New perspectives in clinical microbiology

New perspectives in clinical microbiology

1

Editor
William Brumfitt

Assistant Editor
J.M.T. Hamilton-Miller

1978
Kluwer Medical
Martinus Nijhoff Medical Division

London
The Hague

Contents

Published in Great Britain
and the Commonwealth
by
Kluwer Medical
Forge House
20 Market Place
Brentford
Middlesex TW8 8EQ

in all other
countries
by
Martinus Nijhoff
Medical Division
P.O. Box 442
2501 AX The Hague
The Netherlands

ISBN-13: 978-94-011-7510-4

e-ISBN-13: 978-94-011-7508-1

DOI: 10.1007/978-94-011-7508-1

Contributing authors

DR. S.J.D. BROOKS, M.D., M.R.C.P., Lecturer in Medical Microbiology, Royal Free Hospital (London University), London NW3 2QG.

PROF. W. BRUMFITT, M.D., PH.D., F.R.C.P., F.R.C.PATH., Professor of Medical Microbiology, Royal Free Hospital (London University), London NW3 2QG.

DR. R.T.D. EMOND, F.R.C.P., Consultant Physician, Infectious Diseases Department, Royal Free Hospital, London NW3 2QG.

DR. T.H. FLEWETT, M.D., F.R.C.PATH., M.R.C.P., Regional Virus Laboratory, Birmingham B9 5ST.

DR. J.M.T. HAMILTON-MILLER, PH.D., M.R.C.PATH., Senior Lecturer, Department of Medical Microbiology, Royal Free Hospital (London University), London NW3 2QG.

DR. D. HOBSON, M.D., F.R.C.PATH., Department of Medical Microbiology, University of Liverpool, Liverpool L69 3BX.

PROF. A.V. HOFFBRAND, D.M., F.R.C.P., M.R.C.PATH., Professor of Haematology, Royal Free Hospital (London University), London NW3 2QG.

DR. M.B. PEPYS, PH.D., M.R.C.P., Senior Lecturer in Medicine, Departments of Medicine and Immunology, Royal Postgraduate Medical School, Hammersmith Hospital, Du Cane Road, London W12.

DR. A. PERCIVAL, M.A., M.R.C.PATH., Department of Medical Microbiology, University of Liverpool, Liverpool L69 3BX.

DR. E. REES, M.D., Department of Venereology, University of Liverpool, Liverpool L69 3BX.

DR. A.T. WILLIS, M.D., D.Sc., PH.D., F.R.A.C.P., F.R.C.PATH., Director, Public Health Laboratory, Luton and Dunstable Hospital, Luton LU4 0DZ.

Foreword

If the organizers of the excellent symposium, on which this book is based, had wanted to devise an appropriate dramatic opening they could not have done better than to have the first speaker fail to appear because he was incarcerated in his high security isolation unit caring for a patient suffering from green monkey disease. In his consequently undelivered paper, now published in this book, he understandably dwells a little on the place (both philosophical and physical) of the laboratory in the investigation of highly transmissible infections and this subject characterizes the two themes that run through the chapters of this book: the relative roles of microbiologist and clinician in the investigation and management of infected patients, and the techniques, management and diseases most recently to come under scrutiny.

In addition to some airing of the question (which some of us regard as pressing) as to what degree the microbiologist should be clinical and the clinician microbiological, there is welcome attention by the clinical haematologist and immunologist to humoral and cellular factors in infection that are acknowledged to be crucial but relatively understudied. New looks at old diseases – urinary infections, urethritis and enteritis – and at an old drug, metronidazole, for new indications are all provided by authors who are at the advancing fronts of those subjects. The proceedings, completely updated and revised for this publication, seem to me to have been entirely successful in capturing the stimulation and enjoyment of the excellent and instructive symposium.

FRANCIS O'GRADY T.D., M.D., F.R.C.P., F.R.C.Path
Foundation Professor of Microbiology
University of Nottingham.

Preface

A national symposium was held recently at the Royal Free Hospital School of Medicine to discuss new perspectives in clinical microbiology. This meeting was made possible by the generous support from Beecham Research Laboratories.

Considerable time was spent in constructing the programme in order to cover some of the major growth points in medical microbiology. We were fortunate in assembling a group of speakers who have an international reputation.

Although it was not our original intention to publish, such was the interest generated, as evidenced by applications for places at the meeting being four times oversubscribed, that we asked the speakers to update and expand their talks in a form suitable for publication. As a result of this, and the efficiency of the publishers, the book has not suffered the fate of many multi-author works – many of which are out of date before they appear on the bookshelves.

We are especially grateful to Mr. D. Goodchild of Beecham Research Laboratories, for the burden of organizing the meeting, to Mr. Porter, Mr. Graham and Mr. Duncan of Kluwer Publishing Ltd., who gave us constant support and saw the book safely through the press.

Mrs. Monique Farhi undertook the difficult task of transcribing the discussions and Miss A. Hodson prepared the manuscripts for the printer and compiled the index.

W. BRUMFITT
London 1978

1

Collaboration between the laboratory and the infectious diseases physician

R.T.D. EMOND

Introduction

The complexities of modern medicine have inevitably led to greater specialization with lack of understanding and difficulty in communication between different disciplines. Fortunately there has been a long tradition of mutual sympathy and co-operation between the microbiologist and the infectious diseases physician which, I think, has contributed much to the care of the patient, to the well-being of the community and to the advancement of knowledge. In such company there is little to be gained by walking over common ground and more may be accomplished by wandering through less well-charted territory where difficulties are more likely to be encountered. Before going too far, however, I would like to make a few comments about some familiar landmarks.

The value of blood cultures

We are all familiar with the long-established techniques of blood culture in the investigation of the patient with an unexplained fever but

1

we tend to overlook its value in other circumstances. The detection of bacteria in the blood may provide the essential clue to the nature of meningitis or pneumonia; the unusual severity of an attack of chicken-pox may be explained by growing *Staphylococcus aureus* from the bloodstream.

While blood culture tends to be most rewarding at the height of a fever, positive results may still be obtained when the temperature is normal, especially when the patient is dangerously ill or in a shocked state. In recent years increasing awareness of the importance of anaerobic bacteria ensures that blood is usually cultured anaerobically as well as aerobically. Nevertheless, failure to undertake routine anaerobic culture is still an important reason for negative results in patients after abdominal surgery and perhaps more important in patients with post-abortum or post-partum sepsis where rapid and accurate diagnosis may make all the difference between recovery and disability or even death.

Disputes about blood cultures are a reflection on the degree of understanding between the clinician and the laboratory and both are sometimes at fault. Scrupulous care is essential in both the ward and the laboratory if contamination is to be avoided and optimum results achieved. A high incidence of contaminated bottles should not be regarded as an occasion for mutual recrimination but rather indicate the need for self-assessment and for discussion to ascertain the cause and correct the deficiencies. In this connection it is essential that medical students and junior medical staff should be given careful instruction on the correct techniques and the importance of despatching culture bottles quickly to the laboratory. With anaerobic cultures there is much to be said for the bacteriologist taking the samples himself by the bedside. The experienced clinician will ensure that blood cultures are taken before commencing treatment but all too frequently treatment has already been started before admission to hospital in which case one cannot emphasize too strongly the need to inform the bacteriologist. While most laboratories accept blood cultures without question a few place restrictions on their use. This is somewhat unwise, in my view, for it may not be possible to interpret the significance of a low-grade pathogen in a blood culture unless it has been isolated on several occasions.

Throat swabs

The taking of throat swabs is usually delegated to the nursing staff, some of whom are very experienced and efficient but others move frequently from one hospital or department to another and cannot be relied upon to take the throat swab properly. In such circumstances it behoves the doctor to take the swab himself especially when diphtheria is suspected. Diphtheria, being a rare disease, presents a difficult problem to the bacteriologist. Many junior technicians have never dealt with a wild strain but have practised on stock laboratory organisms which present a classical picture when grown on the usual laboratory media whilst wild strains often do not. Moreover it is difficult to ensure that fresh culture medium is always readily available and that interest is sustained in the routine search for what is now an elusive organism. I feel that the clinician must share the responsibility by alerting the pathologist whenever there is the least suspicion of diphtheria so that an experienced technician can process the specimen.

Examination of faeces

Stool examination can be a tedious chore with so few positive results in relation to the number of patients who appear to have infectious diarrhoea. Even with good facilities it is seldom possible to identify a bacterial pathogen in more than 15-20% of patients with an acute episode of diarrhoea. The recognition of rotaviruses as a cause of gastroenteritis has reduced the number of unexplained cases but we still have far to go (see Chapter 7). I think that our attitude has been too rigid and for too long we have been content to accept 'no pathogens isolated' as a reasonable report when this merely means that culture was negative for salmonellae, shigellae and certain strains of enteropathogenic *Escherichia coli*. Other organisms are discarded as non-pathogenic yet it is difficult to believe that viruses are necessarily responsible for the unexplained cases. Obviously cost and the careful use of resources are important but accurate identification of the causes of infectious diarrhoea is essential if we are to have any hope of elucidating the epidemiology and eradicating the source of infection. Recently the recognition of the role played by some other bacteria (for example *Vibrio parahaemolyticus*, *Bacillus cereus* and *Campylobacter fetus*) in causing food poisoning emphasizes the continuing need for research. Routine culture for cholera vibrios is not reasonable in the United Kingdom or in patients coming from Northern Europe but should always be undertaken in anyone arriving from Asia, Africa or the Mediterranean littoral with diarrhoea of recent onset. The responsibility for requesting the examination should rest with the clinician.

In some laboratories direct microscopy is part of the routine examination of stools; in others it is not and must be specially requested. In my view direct examination is essential in all travellers from abroad with diarrhoea and in residents of the United Kingdom with chronic diarrhoea. In such patients giardiasis is a common cause which will be missed if the diagnosis relies on culture alone. During the past few years we have noted a sharp increase in the number of patients

3

presenting with amoebic abscess of the liver; we have even detected two or three instances where the patient has never been abroad so presumably has been infected from sources within the United Kingdom. The diagnosis has been greatly simplified by modern techniques in liver scanning accompanied by serological tests for *Entamoeba histolytica*.

Positive stool cultures are usually dealt with promptly and results despatched with a sense of urgency. Unfortunately this is not always so with negative findings yet these may be equally important to the community physician or to the patient waiting on tenterhooks for his third 'negative' before discharge or return to work.

Urine culture

Urine culture for evidence of infection can be of considerable importance in the elucidation of a PUO. I have not found urine tests to be of much value in typhoid fever because in the United Kingdom they are seldom positive, either in acute cases of typhoid or in carriers. In patients with septicaemia urine culture may reveal the organism when blood cultures fail and thus enable the all-important sensitivity pattern of the organism to be determined.

Sensitivity testing

Advice on the sensitivity of bacteria to antibiotics is one of the most useful services provided by the laboratory, and guidance on the rational use of these life-saving drugs is one of the areas where the skills of the microbiologist and the infectious diseases physician complement each other. On the whole, antibiotic sensitivity results are of little value in gastrointestinal infections since the common infections often do not benefit from treatment. In contrast the increasing resistance of *Salmonella typhi* in some parts of the world is a cause for concern and indicates the need to determine the sensitivity of this organism as a routine, especially in patients from South-east Asia or Mexico. Similarly the changing pattern of sensitivity of meningococci and gonococci emphasizes the need for vigilance. Of particular value to the physician in recent years has been the facility for testing tubercle bacilli against the wide range of drugs available, enabling him to select those with the least troublesome side-effects. In bacterial endocarditis and in septicaemia rapid identification of the organism and determination of its sensitivity to antibiotics is essential if life is to be saved and damage reduced to a minimum. Monitoring of serum levels of antibiotics to ensure a bactericidal effect is a valuable adjunct and should be performed regularly. Thus facilities for such tests should be available.

Serological tests

Serological tests have been one of the main pillars of diagnosis from the beginnings of microbiology but in recent years these have been eclipsed by the emphasis on isolation and identification of the organism. In my experience the Widal test, in particular, has lost much of its former pre-eminence as a diagnostic aid, partly due to the variation in results for technical reasons and partly from the unpredictable variation in the individual response to infection which makes interpretation of the findings difficult. With all its faults it is still a useful test when cultures prove to be negative and gives authority to the conjectures of the clinician. Brucellosis is a comparatively rare disease in this country but is always considered in the differential diagnosis of the PUO. Blood culture is often disappointing especially in abortus fever and we are all familiar with the patient in whom the disease is strongly suspected but serological tests prove disconcertingly negative. Perhaps the answer lies with research into more sensitive methods of detecting antibodies.

Serological tests come into their own in the context of virus infections where routine culture is usually tedious and expensive. This is particularly true of respiratory virus disease where simple complement-fixation tests on paired sera generally provide an easy retrospective diagnosis. It is less true of virus infections of the bowel and nervous system where routine tests are either not available or involve cumbersome neutralization techniques which prohibit their routine use (but see Chapter 7). In the realm of protozoology, antibody studies have proved to be a great boon in the diagnosis of invasive amoebiasis and in determining the nature of liver abscesses. Unfortunately routine serological tests are not available for the diagnosis of malaria, where reliance is still placed on direct examination of blood smears. Admittedly in skilled hands reliable results are obtained with thick films but difficulties sometimes arise in the management of patients from the tropics with PUO when repeated smears prove negative. This is particularly so when the differential diagnosis rests between Lassa fever or Marburg disease and malaria.

Virology

One of the branches of microbiology which has expanded most in recent years has been virology. As yet there are few safe anti-viral drugs so the main effort has been directed towards accurate diagnosis to establish the pattern of disease and enable control measures to be taken. The results have been truly amazing—the virtual eradication of smallpox from the globe; the elimination of poliomyelitis from much of Europe and North America; the control of yellow fever, and still the

5

critics carp that we cannot cure the common cold! The virologist has already revealed a profusion of different virus infections, many of which are indistinguishable from each other clinically and can only be identified in the laboratory. It is, of course, possible for the experienced physician to make an accurate diagnosis providing the clinical pattern is characteristic and constant. These criteria are met in some of the exanthemata, such as measles, chicken-pox, herpes zoster and smallpox, but even in these conditions diagnosis may be delayed until the characteristic rash emerges. Accurate clinical appraisal is seldom possible with respiratory infections or with generalized infections, as for example cytomegalovirus disease or arbovirus infections. Early and accurate diagnosis may be essential for the control of such infections as smallpox or viral haemorrhagic fevers and for effective chemotherapy should anti-viral drugs prove successful. Electron microscopy has revolutionized the early and prompt diagnosis of smallpox, enabling the clinician and community physician to institute the necessary control measures within a few hours of taking the specimens. In fact pox viruses and herpes viruses with their characteristic shapes and high local concentrations have provided much of the initial stimulus for diagnostic electron microscopy. More recently electron microscopy has unravelled some of the mystery of 'non-specific' gastroenteritis by revealing unsuspected rotaviruses in stools. Immunofluorescent techniques have been bedevilled by lack of sensitivity and have not yet fulfilled their early promise. It seems likely, however, that a combination of electron microscopy and fluorescent techniques may offer the best hope for rapid identification of viruses, especially when anti-viral therapy becomes a practical possibility.

Hepatitis has provided a happy hunting ground for both the immunologist and virologist. The discovery of hepatitis-B antigen and other markers has provided an effective tool for unravelling the epidemiological mysteries of the disease and offer hope of controlling its spread not only in the hospital but in the community. At present the diagnosis of virus A hepatitis is largely a matter of exclusion, and some readily available test is urgently required to enable a positive diagnosis to be made.

The increasing incidence of virus B in hospital patients, particularly among drug addicts, immune-deficient patients and dialysis patients, and the widespread publicity given to outbreaks affecting staff, have made hospitals more safety-conscious. Unfortunately the increasing use of automatic techniques in haematology and biochemistry in conjunction with the large volumes of blood fed into the laboratory by the insatiable demands of modern medicine have enhanced the dangers. Most hospital workers are aware of the risks, and control measures identifying the infected patient and hazardous samples have reaped their rewards. Perhaps we are now too safety-conscious and by denying the antigen-positive patient the benefits of laboratory assessment, as some do, we may be depriving him of the chance of accurate diagnosis and treatment. Of course it is reasonable to take precautions but a balance should be struck between the needs of the individual and the well-being of the community. Surely this is a problem that can be resolved by planning and careful techniques.

Hazards in the laboratory are not a new problem, as many early bacteriologists discovered to their cost, and some pathogens still have a sinister reputation, particularly the agents responsible for tularaemia, psittacosis, tuberculosis and hepatitis B to mention but a few. More recently we have had the spectre of the viral haemorrhagic fevers thrust upon us revealing in the limelight deficiencies in current arrangements. Very few laboratories throughout the world are equipped to process these deadly viruses and routine laboratories have quite understandably been reluctant to handle such dangerous material. This has presented the clinician and the community physician with great problems in establishing the diagnosis in febrile patients from the tropics and makes clinical management of the confirmed case a matter of guesswork. Unfortunately it is not possible on clinical grounds to make an accurate assessment of these patients because there are no characteristic features during the early stages of the illness and the differential diagnosis includes such varied entities as malaria, septicaemia, typhoid fever, acute respiratory virus infections and arbovirus disease. Using a combination of epidemiological evidence and clinical judgement the probabilities can be narrowed down but in most cases accurate diagnosis depends ultimately on the skill of the microbiologist.

The problem is of our own making for, like Oberon, 'we the globe can compass soon swifter than the wandering moon' (Shakespeare) and certainly within the incubation period of most infectious diseases. No region is now remote and the scale of civil engineering projects in rural Africa and the ceaseless quest for oil and other minerals is no longer conducted at a mule's pace but on the swift wings of a company aeroplane. The magnitude of the problem may be gauged from the 100 000 travellers a day passing through Heathrow Airport, not to mention the other major airports serving the South-east of England. From Africa alone over 2200 passengers a day enter London. There is a natural tendency for people to return home when they fall sick abroad and one major airline is aware that it transports more than 500 passengers a year from West Africa suffering from feverish illnesses and no doubt many others travel unrecognized. Since it is impracticable to control or inspect these vast hordes it is inevitable that air travel will resurrect many old plagues and introduce terrifying newcomers creating problems for the clinician, pathologist and community physician alike. It, therefore, behoves all medical practitioners to consider the possibility of an exotic infection in any patient who has recently returned from the tropics, particularly from Africa.

7

Investigation of 'high risk' diseases

Having considered the possibility and admitted the patient to a place of safety the difficulties begin. A sample of blood, a throat swab, urine and faeces are collected, packed securely and despatched by personal messenger to the Microbiological Research Establishment where they are processed in the high-security unit to exclude Lassa fever and Marburg disease. However, a difficult problem remains for the vast majority of these patients will be free from either of these diseases and will be suffering from some other infection. In my experience in the high-security unit of the Royal Free Hospital Infectious Diseases Department about a third of them will have malaria, another third a variety of respiratory virus infections including influenza, and the remainder a pot-pourri of infectious conditions. With malaria a strong possibility and treatment of falciparum infection an urgent necessity, it is imperative to examine blood films for parasites yet it must be conceded that it is hazardous to undertake this in routine laboratories. Unfortunately in an age of laboratory specialization those laboratories with high-security facilities may lack the necessary expertise and delay is inevitable if blood films are to be prepared and then sent to the expert in another laboratory for examination. Admittedly one can always start treatment without waiting for the result but logistics are much simpler if a positive diagnosis can be made within an hour or two and the patient released from the rigours of strict isolation. Similarly haematological, biochemical and other microbiological investigations are essential for the elucidation of a PUO and the management of the patient. While it is acceptable to despatch specimens to a distant reference laboratory for culture of dangerous viruses it is essential that high-security facilities are available locally for other urgent tests. These would include blood smears for malaria, blood cultures for typhoid fever and septicaemia, and simple blood counts. Should the patient recover and the diagnosis remain in doubt the possibility of an arbovirus infection should be considered and an attempt made to establish a retrospective diagnosis by testing paired sera for appropriate antibodies.

Among the complications likely to arise with viral haemorrhagic fevers are disseminated intravascular coagulation, haemorrhage and renal failure. In such circumstances management would be more precise if facilities were readily available for estimating clotting factors, for blood grouping and cross-matching, and for measuring electrolyte levels. Since at present it is not possible to render blood samples safe to examine in the open laboratory it would seem essential to provide a high-security cabinet in which these investigations can be conducted without exposing laboratory workers to risk.

In conclusion I would like to stress how greatly we, in the Infectious Diseases Department, appreciate the skills and knowledge of our colleagues in the laboratory and realize that without their contribution our patients would be the first to suffer and our own professional lives would be that much poorer. I hope, therefore, you will not regard these musings as criticisms but rather as an attempt to identify difficulties which sometimes arise in our joint endeavours to combat infection.

Editor's note

I am most grateful to Dr. Ronald Emond who could not appear at the symposium because he was himself in isolation caring for a patient with Ebola virus infection. Nevertheless, he kindly produced a manuscript rapidly. Clearly there can be no discussion of his paper, but I am most grateful to him for his collaboration. W.B.

2

The role of the laboratory in the control of antimicrobial chemotherapy

A. PERCIVAL

Despite the use of antimicrobial agents for forty years, they are commonly incorrectly and even more often unnecessarily used. In a recent test of knowledge in the United States [1], physicians' mean correct score was 68%. It would not be surprising under stressful conditions (such as the presence of an ill patient) if doctors performed even less well. For example, in a retrospective study [2] in one American hospital, only 13% of antimicrobial therapy given systemically was thought rational, 66% was considered irrational and 22% questionable. Of the irrational treatments half were judged to have been unnecessary and the other half consisted of an inappropriate agent. The commonest indication [2] for the use of antimicrobial agents was prophylaxis (54%).

Current practice in the United Kingdom is unlikely to be any better. I found that 60% of all patients on general medical and surgical wards in one English hospital were given systemic antimicrobial agents during their period in hospital and, in 70% of them, there was no established indication stated in the case notes or justified by results of microbiological investigations (unpublished observations). In domiciliary practice, the situation is even less satisfactory, although the reasons for prescribing may be more compelling. For example, 60 of 100 babies attending a local clinic had received at least one course of antibiotics during the first year of life, usually broad-spectrum, and for trivial reasons such as teething, runny nose, nappy rash and diarrhoea. Not once had a diagnostic specimen been sent for microbiological examination.

All such observations expose the limited extent to which antimicrobial therapy has been and can perhaps ever be influenced by laboratory guidance. Laboratories, too, make errors, issuing incorrect and, probably more often, irrelevant sensitivity results, and may also be guilty of unjustifiable delays in reporting. However, it is against the background of abuse and misuse of antimicrobial therapy that the routine diagnostic service laboratory ought realistically to consider how best to concentrate its efforts, at a time in this country of increasing workload and financial stringency. This does not deny the legitimate interests of a minority of more specialized laboratories to pursue various aspects of antimicrobial therapy in depth and detail. Nevertheless, the extent to which further refinements and automation of techniques should be generally introduced and have priority of stretched resources needs careful consideration in the light of known therapeutic efficacy and the reluctance of clinicians to change their prescribing habits. If far reaching laboratory changes are to be made their practical value must first be established.

Factors determining the efficacy of antimicrobial agents

Those factors of known or potential importance in determining the efficacy of antimicrobial treatment are shown in Table 1. It is beyond the scope of this chapter to try to review all of these, but it must be emphasized that the traditional area of greatest laboratory involvement, sensitivity testing, is only one of many factors. Clearly, the susceptibility of the infecting organism is of fundamental importance but a variety of other factors such as mode of administration, potential toxicity, history of allergy and patient's condition have also to be considered in choosing appropriate therapy. This cannot be done by the laboratory worker without knowledge of all the clinical circumstances.

Sensitivity

The definition of sensitivity is not arbitrary but must relate to the expectation of successful treatment in infected patients—and not mere laboratory tests. Traditionally the word is used in different ways in different clinical situations. Whereas a 'penicillin-resistant' gonococcus (MIC 0.125 to 1 μg/ml) may not be eradicated by a single

---

Table 1. Antimicrobial efficacy depends on:

ORGANISM   — Sensitivity
                 — Rate of division
                 — Numbers present
                 — Production of inactivators

HOST   — State of defences
                 — Site of infection
                 — Pathological factors

DRUG   — Levels (at site)
                 — Duration of exposure
                 — Penetration
                 — Binding
                 — Mode and speed of action
                 — Potentiation or inactivation by milieu or other agents

---

particular dose of benzylpenicillin or ampicillin, but will be by twice that dose, another organism with equivalent sensitivity (e.g. *Haemophilus influenzae* or *Streptococcus faecalis*) is regarded as sensitive because a seven-day course of treatment with similar, multiple doses will be effective. *Pseudomonas aeruginosa* is reported as carbenicillin-sensitive when the MIC is relatively great (50 μg/ml) but an infection by such an organism will be cured only if high-dosage therapy is used (20 to 30 g per day). An organism reported as tetracycline-resistant and causing a superficial skin infection might well respond to topical application of a 2% ointment. Thus, a particular level of *in vitro* susceptibility has different clinical implications for different antibiotics, different organisms and different body sites and must be related to dosage, accessibility and potential toxicity. Therefore, it is essential that clinical and laboratory staff understand each other and it is desirable that laboratory reports should always be made bearing these various relevant factors in mind. This requires a much wider knowledge and understanding than of mere technique. The extent to which quantification of more precise degrees of sensitivity may be of therapeutic significance is considered later. Conventionally, a sensitive organism is regarded as one which is inhibited or killed *in vitro* by an amount of antibiotic which can readily be achieved in the blood of patients and maintained, without toxicity, at several times higher than the MIC for most of the period between doses. The normal dose of an antimicrobial is, therefore, chosen from susceptibility and pharmacological data and has to be verified by clinical trial.

Rate of bacterial division and numbers present

The more slowly dividing pathogens are usually associated with chronic lesions, for example tuberculosis, actinomycosis or fungal infections. These have long been shown to require a relatively prolonged period of treatment but do not necessarily respond only to bactericidal agents. For speed and simplicity, sensitivity tests traditionally are performed in media which encourage rapid growth and need not necessarily reflect the condition at an infected site. Bacteria that are not multiplying may be insusceptible to bactericidal agents, particularly those which act upon the cell wall. After treatment, either a minority of such 'persisters' [3] or cell-wall-free forms (spheroplasts) could cause relapse if protected from the body defence mechanisms in avascular tissue or close to a foreign body. In such infections, some physicians consider it justifiable to use combinations, usually of two different agents which exert *in vitro* a synergistic effect, in that the combination may produce a complete kill of a large inoculum not achieved by either drug alone. The concept seems valid if it can be shown by clinical trial that suitable combinations are more successful in these conditions than single agents.

In the great majority of established infections, the numbers of bacteria in the infected areas are considerable, exceeding 10^5 per ml and often reaching 10^7 per ml in infected urine, homogenised infected sputum or pus. Rationally, a similar inoculum ought to be used in sensitivity tests but there is a growing tendency in MIC determinations with multiple inoculators to employ smaller numbers (10^4 per ml). With most antimicrobial agents, there is usually a two- to fourfold increase in sensitivity with the small inoculum.

Production of inactivators

By 1950, there had been a rapid increase in prevalence of β-lactamase producing *Staphylococcus aureus* in hospitals. Extensive clinical experience of failure of penicillin treatment in infections caused by these organisms understandably resulted in the simple approach that β-lactamase-producing organisms were always to be regarded as resistant to benzylpenicillin. The therapeutically successful introduction of semi-synthetic penicillins resistant to the action of staphylococcal β-lactamase and, subsequently, a very considerable increase in knowledge of the great variety of different β-lactamases widespread among numerous bacteria, has created a much more complicated situation. Furthermore, new penicillins and cephalosporins with varying degrees of susceptibility to different β-lactamases continue to be introduced.

Sensitive techniques such as iso-electric focusing using a chromogenic cephalosporin [4] as indicator for β-lactamase have revealed that perhaps every bacterium possesses at least a minor degree of this enzyme activity. Much is known of the role that the enzymes play in determining susceptibility to penicillins and cephalosporins *in vitro* and this is admirably reviewed elsewhere [5], but far less is established for the *in vivo* situation. Mere traces of the enzyme activity are apparently present even in pathogenic bacteria highly sensitive to benzylpenicillin and ampicillin and must therefore be of little therapeutic importance. For example, small amounts of β-lactamase activity were observed in strains of *Escherichia coli* [6] from patients with acute pyelonephritis who were successfully treated with normal doses of ampicillin. When production of the enzyme is determined by plasmids, as in staphylococci and some Gram-negative bacteria, relatively large amounts of enzyme are made, particularly if it is inducible.

In addition, the acquisition of plasmids by pathogenic bacteria such as *H. influenzae* [7] and gonococci [8] from other bacterial species by conjugation [9-11] is a growing problem and likely to continue. Perhaps β-lactamase-producing meningococci or other bacteria will emerge. In gonococci, the β-lactamase certainly is responsible for failure to respond not only to single doses but also to 5 and 10 day regimens of penicillins which are susceptible to the enzymes [8]. Also β-lactamase producing strains of *H. influenzae*, have been associated with failure of meningitis to be cured by large doses of ampicillin [12]. With organisms which are innately relatively sensitive to penicillins (staphylococci, gonococci, *H. influenzae*), strains producing easily recognizable quantities of β-lactamase show a marked inoculum effect in sensitivity tests. This may be missed unless inocula exceeding 10^5 per ml are used. In organisms with a greater permeability barrier to penicillins through the cell wall, for example enterobacteria, only relatively small quantities of β-lactamase are sufficient to confer appreciable resistance *in vitro* [6] and there is much less inoculum effect in sensitivity tests. In my experience, the same is found with bacteria which inactivate aminoglycosides enzymatically. It has been suggested that even minor differences in stability to β-lactamase are important in deciding the choice of a particular penicillin or cephalosporin for general use [13, 14] but, as yet, this is not supported by any clinical evidence. Thus, the implications for the laboratory are perplexing, not only as to which agents to test and in what manner, but also how to justify any definite recommendations.

Host factors

Details of previous history of allergy, site and nature of the lesion, current or recent antimicrobial therapy, feasibility of a particular mode of administration, and body weight are all relevant in deciding which agent to give and at what dosage. The concept of a normal dose is, perhaps, unfortunate because it often seems to inhibit considerations of the patient's individual circumstances. Impairment in function of an excretory organ, especially the kidney, is particularly important if toxicity is to be avoided. All should be known before a laboratory advises in a difficult individual problem, although not necessary for routine sensitivity reports. Diminished body defences, either locally or generally, may influence choice of treatment and its duration. Obstruction is generally accepted as a major cause of difficulty in treatment, in part at least because of both reduced wash-out effect and lowered concentration of antimicrobial in the drainage system from obstructed excretory organs. Failure of conventional treatment may often be the first indication of this type of underlying abnormality.

Penetration of drug to and activity at site of infection

Apart from topical application or local instillation, the antimicrobial has to reach the site of infection from the blood stream. It has long been known that concentration by excretion from the liver and kidneys leads to levels in the biliary and urinary tracts, of some agents, greatly exceeding those in the blood. In contrast, most antimicrobial agents do not penetrate well into the CSF or sputum, where at best the levels achieved are lower than in the blood. In recent years, renewed attention has been paid to studies on penetration into the tissues. This is difficult to estimate because measurements on homogenates may merely reflect the amount of blood or excretory fluid in the material, whilst attempts to wash out the blood beforehand may lead to loss from the tissues of rapidly diffusing antibiotics. Consequently, attempts have been made to simulate tissue fluid in implanted plastic 'cages' [15] or by skin abrasion [16, 17] and to assay levels in lymph [18] and various exudates [19-21]. Again, all these and earlier studies on pus [22] show that peak levels are reached later, are much lower but tend to persist longer than in the blood. In prostatic secretions, the great majority of antimicrobial agents never reach inhibitory levels [23].

Excluding the role played by the natural defences, the implications are that perhaps peak blood levels grossly overestimate tissue concentrations but that the latter fluctuate much less during the conventional multiple dose regimens. Therefore, for all but the most susceptible micro-organisms, the margin between tissue concentrations and sensitivity apparently is a narrow one. In designing sensitivity tests, the laboratory should bear this in mind where appropriate and take care, for example in disc testing, not to use amounts of antibiotic which are too high. For the same reason, therapy of life-threatening infections with potentially toxic antimicrobial agents is now thought by some to require monitoring the blood levels in each patient. The need is accentuated by marked individual variation in blood levels after a particular dose, even when it has been carefully given by intravenously 'bolus' injection in order to exclude poor injection technique and irregular absorption from injection sites as contributory factors. All studies on sputum levels show an even greater individual variation, not explained by differences in the inflammatory exudative component.

It is clear that factors determining the passage of antimicrobials into tissue fluids and exudates (molecular size, pK, lipid solubility, binding to tissues and plasma proteins) are of varying importance for different tissues and such passage cannot be explained solely in terms of simple diffusion.

The role of plasma protein binding is not clear and has probably been over emphasized. The highly bound antibiotics, fusidic acid and cloxacillin, have not consistently shown low levels in the studies on tissue penetration, and are therapeutically effective, for example in osteomyelitis, even when blood levels of unbound antibiotic could not have been inhibitory. In addition, binding by tissues [24] is another independent factor at least of theoretically equal significance.

Local conditions at the site of infection can affect antimicrobial activity, for example when it is significantly pH-dependent [25]. Recently, inactivation of penicillins and cephalosporins by pus has been described in a patient with empyema [26] who failed to respond to penicillin treatment and in 4 of 22 specimens examined by others [27]. This was not due to β-lactamase or pH effect but was thought to be enzyme-mediated. The reason why only certain specimens had this property remains to be discovered but the observation potentially provides the laboratory with much future work in the investigation of individual treatment failures. Inactivation of trimethoprim by thymidine in pus can readily be demonstrated *in vitro* [28] but its possible clinical significance has yet to be shown. Reversal of the activity of the sulphonamides by para-aminobenzoic acid including that preformed in a large bacterial inoculum has long been known but sulphonamides remain highly effective therapeutic agents against infections caused by sensitive organisms.

17

Mode and speed of action of drug and duration of exposure to it

Speculations as to the relative merits of bactericidal or bacteriostatic agents continue with renewed vigour following the observations [29-31] that 'tolerant' strains of *Staph. aureus* inhibited but only killed at very much higher concentrations by penicillins or cephalosporins were not uncommon among isolates from severe infections. If these infections could be clearly shown not to respond adequately to treatment with β-lactamase-stable penicillins or cephalosporins, laboratory tests of bactericidal effect may be routinely needed for bacteria known to be capable of such behaviour. These findings provide one explanation of the synergistic effects of combinations of bactericidal agents and their strain to strain variation. Perhaps tests of combined action also will now be needed more commonly.

However, it should be remembered that bacteriostatic drugs have already proved to be very effective in the great majority of infections and even single doses of tetracyclines eradicate highly sensitive gonococci from 90% of patients [32]. In addition, in the frequently severe condition of bacteraemia caused by Gram-negative rods, bacteriostatic agents were as effective as bactericidal ones in patients without underlying disease likely to be fatal within six months [33]. Unfortunately, in the study, the numbers of patients investigated likely to have generalized impairment of body defences and to benefit from bactericidal therapy, were too few for comparison. The problem is unlikely to be resolved by clinical trial because of the ethical difficulties invoked in treating life-threatening infections with agents theoretically thought to be inferior.

Relatively more subtle differences between the speeds and detailed modes of the bactericidal actions of different β-lactam drugs (amoxycillin, mecillinam and cephalosporins) are currently employed in some promotion literature. Also, they are a basis for microbiologists' continued preoccupations with inoculum size, effects of media content and osmolality, persistence of cell-wall-free forms, whether turbidity profiles have greater relevance than traditional MIC determinations [34] and the possible advantages of various combinations. Meanwhile, potential users of these various competing but essentially similar antibiotics presumably look on in confused bewilderment whilst reported clinical trials have yet to suggest any significant therapeutic differences.

Current practice is toward reduction in periods of antimicrobial therapy. In domiciliary patients, treatment with amoxycillin for 3 days was as successful as for 10 [35], and acceptable results have been achieved in streptococcal endocarditis after only two weeks' treatment with penicillin and streptomycin [36]. A relevant consideration is whether the aim is to bring about symptomatic relief, to ensure complete eradication of the organism or to achieve prophylactic suppression, the site of infection being of great importance [37]. A few days' treatment with benzylpenicillin will relieve a streptococcal sore throat but injections for 10 days are needed to eradicate the organism [38]. Equally, sensitive meningococci and gonococci are also difficult to remove from the throat but a single dose of benzylpenicillin will eradicate gonococci from the cervix and rectum of 95% of infected women.

Interdependence

Many of the various factors affecting antimicrobial efficacy clearly are interrelated and therefore difficult to assess in the infected patient or even an animal model. For both clinician and microbiologist, there exists an ever-increasing number of similar antimicrobial agents with different br and proper names. For most infections the choice is too great and confusing. Many of the *in vitro* studies already mentioned create pressures upon the laboratory for additional and more complicated time consuming work to explore antimicrobial therapy in greater depth. However, apart from increasing problems due to resistance, bacterial infections continue to be effectively treated in the majority of patients and the great majority of viral infections resolve spontaneously. In searching for reasons for failure of treatment, it has also to be remembered that bacterial toxins and mechanical or embolic complications may have fatal effects despite and after institution of adequate antimicrobial therapy.

Laboratory guidance – susceptibility testing

Sensitivities

The important aspects are summarized in Table 2. Sensitivity tests should only be reported for organisms likely to be of clinical significance, requiring and expected to benefit from antimicrobial therapy. This may be difficult to judge from within the laboratory but, when there is uncertainty, a suitable compromise is to perform the tests and report 'sensitivities available on request'. For example, *Klebsiella aerogenes* from sputum of a patient receiving ampicillin is unlikely to be more than part of a secondary throat flora unless persistently present in large numbers in purulent material. The decision whether to treat or not will then depend on that patient's clinical and radiological progress and can be guided by asking the laboratory for the withheld information. Also *Pseudomonas* spp. in a varicose ulcer or bed sore is best treated by topical agents not used for systemic therapy. Withholding sensitivities on 'second line' antimicrobial agents may contribute to hospital policies for antibiotic use but our practice is always to test a relatively wide range in order to avoid delay when isolates prove to be multiply resistant.

Sensitivities should only be reported to relevant antimicrobial agents and not, for example, to nitrofurantoin for *Esch. coli* from pus or to ampicillin for *Strept. pyogenes* from the throat. Incorporation of

---

Table 2. Laboratory guidance in antimicrobial chemotherapy — susceptibility testing

SENSITIVITIES   — Relevant organisms
— Related to usual therapy
— Correct technically
— Correct interpretation
— Tests for inactivators a useful adjunct

PRECISION REQUIRED (MICs)
Life-threatening infections, treated by relatively toxic agents or due to relatively resistant organisms
Response known to be critically dose dependent

---

certain agents into multiple sensitivity tests may have other uses within a laboratory as an aid to identification and for purposes of monitoring resistance trends but need not be reported to the clinician.

The sensitivity report must relate to 'usual' therapeutic dosage, assuming that laboratory and clinician agree as to what this is. Misunderstandings seem to occur particularly when terms such as 'sensitive only to high dosage' or even less explicit, 'moderately sensitive' or 'partially resistant' are used. Probably of greatest importance in paper-disc testing is the choice of an appropriate amount of antibiotic to be incorporated into the disc. The greatest and potentially most serious mistake is of an incorrect report indicating sensitivity and is the main disadvantage of using high disc content in order to recognise degrees of susceptibility. The commonest bad error, in my experience, has been *Staph. aureus* recorded as resistant to benzyl penicillin (1-μg disc) but sensitive to ampicillin (25-μg disc). Previously, we found that pneumococci resistant to tetracycline (MICs 10 to 25 μg/ml) were not identified with 50-μg but were by 10-μg discs [39]. Recently, we have observed that 10-μg discs do not discriminate gonococci with MICs of 2-4 μg/ml from more sensitive strains but the former are associated with significantly more treatment failures [8, 40]. The strength of nitrofurantoin discs should be such (50 μg) that only small inhibitory zones are obtained with *Proteus* spp. from urinary tract infections which do not respond to treatment with this agent, but zones with *Esch. coli* should be appreciable (20 mm in diameter or more) [41].

False reports of resistance, though less dangerous, are probably commoner, especially with the more inoculum-dependent agents such as sulphonamides and trimethoprim. These cause confusion in judging the sequence of events in individual patients, for example whether there is relapse or re-infection and may limit the use of valuable therapeutic agents by creating an incorrect impression of high prevalance of resistant organisms.

During a recent qualifying examination for microbiology technicians, it was disturbing to find that in answering a question on factors affecting sensitivity testing by paper disc, 70% did not mention the two most important; disc strength and sensitivity of the tested organism. On the other hand, many of the others, depth, pH, magnesium content and type of medium, inoculum size, pre-diffusion, presence of inactivators were well reviewed. Quality-control studies [42] have revealed a disquieting incidence of false reporting and is still common in this country. The long recognized problem areas continue to provide the most discrepancies, sulphonamide, trimethoprim and co-trimoxazole, methicillin-resistant staphylococci and the problem of testing carbenicillin against pseudomonas. Thus, at a time when recent pressures are in favour of more sophisticated laboratory techniques in control of antimicrobial therapy, many diagnostic laboratories are still unable to carry out the relatively simple tests correctly.

Errors of interpretation rather than of technique appear to be more frequent. Controlled tests [43, 44] against standard organisms certainly reveal those discs which contain no antibiotic or have lost activity during storage. However, interpretation may become more confused unless appropriate standard organisms are used, for example when comparing *H. influenzae* or *Strept. faecalis* with the highly sensitive Oxford staphylococcus.

Tests for inactivators

A simple rapid test of β-lactamase production is a useful adjunct to sensitivity testing. A loopful of culture is spread on to a drop of chromogenic cephalosporin [45] on filter paper and a red colour change produced by β-lactamase. This test distinguishes between β-lactamase-producing strains of certain species, *H. influenzae*, gonococci and *Proteus mirabilis* which should be reported as benzylpenicillin or ampicillin resistant. However, it does not help with other bacterial species in which sufficient constitutive enzyme to produce a positive result is present in all strains. (For example, *Esch. coli*, *Klebsiella* spp., *Pseudomonas* spp., *Bacteroides fragilis*.) A similar test for aminoglycoside-inactivating enzymes would be helpful.

Precision required

More precise determination of sensitivity is needed for life-threatening infections treated by relatively toxic agents such as the aminoglycosides because the margin between effective but potentially toxic therapy is a narrow one. Since successful therapy with gentamicin was significantly reduced when peak blood levels did not exceed 8 μg/ml [46], it follows that relatively insusceptible organisms (MICs 8–12 μg/ml) need to be recognized. The same is true for other infections where response is known to be critically dose dependent, for example, streptococcal endocarditis. Our experience with tetracycline and gonococci, already mentioned, suggests that this requirement may well be commoner than has hitherto been recognized. Further clinical studies relating response to degree of sensitivity are necessary to explore the possibility.

Special circumstances

Indications for laboratory tests additional to those concerned with antimicrobial susceptibility are summarized in Table 3. There has been

---

Table 3. Laboratory guidance in antimicrobial chemotherapy — special circumstances

BLOOD LEVELS REQUIRED
    When effective but potentially toxic levels close
    For continued oral therapy of serious infections

TESTS FOR SYNERGISTIC COMBINATIONS
    Endocarditis by relatively insensitive organisms

ADVICE ON FAILURE TO RESPOND TO TREATMENT

OTHER FACTORS MUST BE CONSIDERED
    Aim—eradication or control
    Allergy, administration, patient condition, potential toxicity, etc.

---

an explosion in the technology related to the determination of aminoglycoside blood levels and this is reviewed elsewhere [47]. Quality control programmes have again shown a disturbingly high incidence of 'misleading' results although the degree of accuracy required for therapeutic success is a source of dispute. It is argued by some that a 25% discrepancy may be acceptable. Nevertheless, differences between peak plasma levels of 6 and 8 μg/ml could be of therapeutic significance and between trough levels of 2 and 3 μg/ml relevant to potential toxicity. Unfortunately, the more precise methods require expensive equipment.

When employing oral therapy for serious infections, for example endocarditis with penicillins, estimation of blood levels is mandatory to confirm that adequate absorption occurs. Experience with actinomycosis indicates that the same applies in that condition and future studies may well extend the indications.

Tests for synergistic combinations are of established value in endocarditis caused by relatively resistant organisms, staphylococci, *Strept. faecalis* and fungi, and are described elsewhere [48]. Other difficult infections, fungal [49], chronic osteomyelitis and those associated with implants or prostheses, may benefit from combined therapy designed by laboratory tests of synergy.

The laboratory can help in a variety of ways to advise on failure to respond to treatment. Blood-level determinations will reveal whether dosage and absorption are adequate and the patient's blood or exudates can be used to see if they are inhibitory or bactericidal against the infecting organism. If they are, then a penetration problem exists and may indicate the need for surgical intervention. If they are not, dosage needs to be increased or treatment changed. Specialized further investigations can be recommended to exclude or confirm the presence of another or different causative organism. The clinically orientated microbiologist can also recommend correction of inappropriate therapy and perhaps recognize that apparent treatment failure is not, in fact, due to lack of antimicrobial control but to other disease processes or complications of the therapy itself. Thus, we return to the limitations imposed when advice is offered only from within the laboratory without a visit to see the patient and the opportunity to seek 'first hand' information.

Laboratory involvement in antimicrobial therapy

The laboratory has an essential role to play as a source of advice and guidance to the clinical services. Some or most of these inevitably find increasing difficulty in maintaining sufficient knowledge and expertise in this ever more complicated subject. Areas of legitimate involvement are listed in Table 4. The need for antibiotic policies to ensure more rational use and to limit unnecessary administration is widely acknowledged but little practised. Because of the alarming growth in

Table 4.   Laboratory guidance in antimicrobial chemotherapy—overall involvement

ANTIBIOTIC POLICIES — Choice of agent, proscription, rotation, guidance booklets

MONITORING USE — Overall (pharmacy records)
— Individual patients
— Misuse

RESISTANCE PROBLEMS — Adequate records
— Cross-infection control

resistant organisms, particularly in hospitals, such policies are urgently needed. Guidance pocket-sized booklets provide a helpful source of ready-to-hand information, but tend to be produced by only a few individual hospitals. None is commercially available. A crucial part of any control is the pharmacy, which should maintain and periodically produce six-monthly records of overall use. From these, areas and instances of misuse can be recognized. Contact with clinicians about individual patients or particular practices is also necessary, but as doctors wish to retain their prescribing rights the help of clinicians in defining an antibiotic policy is apparent.

Each laboratory should keep its own records of resistance trends. These should include common cross-infecting organisms such as *Staph. aureus* and pseudomonads or any other locally prevalent organisms, any instances of newly emerged resistance and all resistance to important reserve or 'last-line' antimicrobial agents. *Staph. aureus* resistant to gentamicin or methicillin or gentamicin resistant bacteria in a lesion is an indication for containment isolation of the patient before spread occurs to others. The lack of any significant increase in resistance of *M. tuberculosis* to antituberculous agents is an encouraging example of what can be achieved when the importance of the problem is generally accepted by those involved.

Recent trends

Recent trends in involvement and preoccupations of laboratories in antimicrobial chemotherapy, technically and conceptually, are summarized in Table 5. Some have already been discussed.

Table 5. Recent trends in laboratory control of antimicrobial therapy

TECHNIQUE — Controlled sensitivity testing
— More precise sensitivity testing
— More blood-level determinations
— Quality control
— Automation
— Data processing and retrieval

CONCEPT — Effects of antibiotics at concentrations less than the MIC
— Sequential actions
— Differences in dynamics and details of mode of action
— Role of inactivators
— Variation in differences between MIC and MBC

Automation

Automation is an established and integral part of the chemical pathology and haematology laboratories whilst microbiology lags behind. However, automation in microbiology is now possible and susceptibility testing is a promising field [50]. For the small laboratory, disposable plastic trays primed with freeze-dried antibiotic dilutions offer a satisfactory means of MIC determination and it is to be hoped that the choice of combinations and range of dilutions of antimicrobials available will soon be widened. Other methods all involve the purchase of expensive equipment but offer the possibilities of more rapid and more precise results than disc-diffusion tests, although these can be read the same day with many more rapidly growing pathogens and can be made more precise by using two or three discs of different strengths of the same antibiotic. Since therapy will continue to be initiated 'blind', speed in terms of a few hours is perhaps not generally essential, but labour saving and precision are desirable. Among the difficulties involved, are the different criteria which will need to be evaluated since most machines use optical sensors as growth indicators over a relatively short incubation period and therefore measure changes in bacterial shape and mass rather than viability. Also, these changes occur at concentrations of antimicrobial agents below those obtained in conventional MIC determinations. However, the recognition of antimicrobial effects at such levels is not new [51] and any limitation of microbial growth may be sufficient to allow body

25

defence mechanisms to resolve an infection. A consequence of these developments has been a renewed interest in the study of the effect of concentration of antimicrobial agents below the MIC, [52, 53], which has relevance to the whole question of what constitutes an effective concentration of antibiotic at the site of infection and the consequent criterion of sensitivity. Until verified by clinical observation a reliance on subinhibitory concentrations remains potentially dangerous, not least because therapeutic responses have correlated well with traditional sensitivity tests and MIC determinations [33, 39, 41, 54-58]. For the moment, the value and cost-effectiveness of automatic sensitivity testing needs further evaluation but a determined effort should be made by microbiologists in this country to pursue it and thereby disturb the traditional monopoly held by other sub-specialities of pathology of funds for expensive equipment.

Combined and sequential activities

Despite the limited indications thought to justify the need for antibiotic combinations [59], further possibilities continue to be explored by *in vitro* studies [60, 61] and co-trimoxazole has now been widely used for many years. Unfortunately, such combinations complicate the work of the laboratory in susceptibility testing and lead to confusion between interpretation of actual results and reporting policy. It has been suggested that co-trimoxazole should not be given for infections caused by organisms which are sulphonamide resistant, and some laboratories, therefore, incorrectly report such organisms as co-trimoxazole resistant. This kind of practice can only heighten lack of confidence by clinicians in the diagnostic service. It is dishonest actually to alter results to fit in with a prescribing policy.

Finally, *in vitro* observations have indicated that a type of sequential synergy can occur when organisms damaged by agents acting on the cell wall are thereafter exposed to antimicrobial agents with a different mode of action. For example, erythromycin may have greater activity on spheroplasts induced by penicillins than on the undamaged bacteria. The therapeutic implications remain unexplored.

References

1. Neu, H.C., and Howrey, S.P. (1975) Testing the physician's knowledge of antibiotic use. *New Engl. J. Med.* **293**, 1291–5.
2. Roberts, A.W., and Visconti, J.A. (1972) The rational and irrational use of systemic antimicrobial drugs. *Am. J. Hosp. Pharm.* **29**, 828–34.
3. Bigger, J.H. (1944) Treatment of Staphylococcal infections with penicillin. *Lancet* **ii**, 497–500.

4. Matthew, M., Harris, A.M., Marshall, M.J., and Ross, G.W. (1975) The use of analytical isoelectric focusing for detection and identification of β-lactamases. *J. Gen. Microbiol.* **88**, 169–78.

5. Sykes, R.B., and Matthew, M. (1976) The β-lactamases of Gram-negative bacteria and their role in resistance to β-lactam antibiotics. *J. Antimicrob. Chemother.* **2**, 115–57.

6. Percival, A., Brumfitt, W., and de Louvois, J. (1963) The role of penicillinase in determining natural and acquired resistance of Gram-negative bacteria to penicillins. *J. Gen. Microbiol.* **32**, 77–89.

7. Williams, J.D., and Cavanagh, P. (1974) Ampicillin-resistant *Haemophilus influenzae* meningitis. *Lancet* i, 864.

8. Percival, A., Corkhill, J.E., Arya, O.P., Rowlands, J., Alergant, C.D., Rees, E., and Annels, E.H. (1976) Penicillinase-producing gonococci in Liverpool. *Lancet* ii, 1379–82.

9. Sykes, R.B., Matthew, M., and O'Callaghan, C.H. (1975) R-factor mediated β-lactamase production by *Haemophilus influenzae*. *J. Med. Microbiol.* **8**, 437–41.

10. Roberts, M., and Falkow, S. (1977) Conjugal transfer of R plasmids in *Neisseria gonorrhoea*. *Nature, Lond.* **266**, 630–1.

11. Eisenstein, B.I., Sox, T., Biswas, G., Blackman, E., and Sparling, P.F. (1977) Conjugal transfer of the gonococcal penicillinase plasmid. *Science, N.Y.* **195**, 998–1000.

12. Thomas, W.J., McReynolds, J.W., Mock, C.R., and Bailey, D. (1974) Ampicillin-resistant *Haemophilus influenzae* meningitis. *Lancet* i, 313.

13. Lacey, R.W., and Stokes, A. (1977) Susceptibility of the 'penicillinase-resistant' penicillins and cephalosporins to penicillinase of *Staphylococcus aureus*. *J. Clin. Path.* **30**, 35–9.

14. Selwyn, S. (1976) Rational choice of penicillins and cephalosporins based on parallel *in vitro* and *in vivo* tests. *Lancet* ii, 616–18.

15. Chisholm, G.D., Waterworth, P.M., Calnan, J.S., and Garrod, L.P. (1973) Concentration of antibacterial agents in interstitial tissue fluid. *Br. med. J.* **1**, 569–73.

16. Raeburn, J.A. (1971) A method for studying antibiotic concentrations in inflammatory exudate. *J. clin. Path.* **24**, 633–5.

17. Tan, J.S., Trott, A., Phair, J.P., and Wataukunakorn, C. (1972) A method for measurement of antibiotics in human interstitial fluid. *J. infect. Dis.* **126**, 492–7.

18. Chisholm, G.D., Calnan, J.S., and Waterworth, P.M. (1968) Antibacterial agents in renal lymph. In *Urinary tract infection*. Eds. O'Grady, F., and Brumfitt, W. Oxford University Press, pp. 194–211.

19. Nelson, J.D. (1971) Antibiotic concentrations in septic joint effusions. *New Engl. J. Med.* **284**, 349–53.

20. Nelson, C.L., Bergfeld, J.A., Schwarz, J., and Kokzun, M. (1975) Antibiotics in human haematoma and wound fluid. *Clin. Orthop.* **108**, 138–44.

21. Ellis, B.W., Starbridge, R. de L., Sikorski, J.M., Dudley, H.A.F., and Spencer, R.C. (1975) Penetration into inflammatory exudate and wounds of two cephalosporins for the prevention of surgical infections. *J. Antimicrob. Chemother.* **1**, 291–6.

22. Florey, M.E., Turton, E.C., and Duthie, E.S. (1946) Penicillin in wound exudates. *Lancet* ii, 405–9.

23. Winningham, D.G., Nemoy, N.J., and Stamey, T.A. (1968) Diffusion of antibiotics from plasma into prostatic fluid. *Nature, Lond.* **219**, 139–42.

24. Kunin, C.M. (1970) Binding of antibiotics to tissue homogenates. *J. infect. Dis.* **121**, 55–64.

25. Brumfitt, W., and Percival, A. (1962) Adjustment of urine pH in the chemotherapy of urinary tract infection. *Lancet* i, 186–90.

26. Barnes, P., and Waterworth, P.M. (1977) New cause of penicillin treatment failure. *Br. med. J.* **1**, 991–3.
27. de Louvois, J., and Hurley, R. (1977) Inactivation of penicillin by purulent exudates. *Br. med. J.* **1**, 998–1000.
28. Lacey, R.W. (1976) Antibiotic tissue levels. *Abbott Intake* 44.
29. Best, G.K., Best, N.H., and Koval, A.V. (1974) Evidence for participation of autolysins in bactericidal action of oxacillin on *Staphylococcus aureus*. *Antimicrob. Agents Chemother.* **6**, 825–30.
30. Sabath, L.D., Wheeler, N., Laverdiere, M., Blazevic, D., and Wilkinson, B.J. (1977) A new type of penicillin resistance of *Staphylococcus aureus*. *Lancet* i, 443–7.
31. Mayhall, C.G., Medoff, G., and Marr, J.T. (1976) Variation in susceptibility of strains of *Staphylococcus aureus* to oxacillin, cephalothin and gentamicin. *Antimicrob. Agents Chemother.* **10**, 707–12.
32. McLone, D.G., Billings, T.E., Hardegrie, W.E., and Hackney, J.F. (1968) Gonorrhoea in females treated with one oral dose of tetracycline *Br. J. vener. Dis.* **44**, 218–19.
33. MacCabe, W.R. (1975) Antibiotics and endotoxic shock. *Bull. N.Y. Acad. Med.* **51**, 1084–95.
34. Greenwood, D. (1976) Unrealistic nature of the M.I.C. *J. antimicrob. Chemother.* **2**, 312–13.
35. Charlton, C.A., Crowther, A., Davies, J.G., Dynes, J., Haward, M.W.A., Mann, P.G., and Rye, S. (1976) Three-day and ten-day chemotherapy for urinary tract infections in general practice. *Br. med. J.* **1**, 124–6.
36. Tan, J.S., Terhune, C.A., Kaplan, S., and Hamburger, M. (1971) Successful two-week treatment schedule for penicillin-susceptible *Streptococcus viridans* endocarditis. *Lancet* ii, 1340–3.
37. Angel, J.H. (1977) Short-course chemotherapy in pulmonary tuberculosis. *J. antimicrob. Chemother.* **3**, 290–4.
38. Wannamaker, L.N., Denny, F.W., Perry, W., Rammelkamp, C.H., Eckhardt, G.C., Houser, H.B., and Hahn, E.O. (1953) The effect of penicillin prophylaxis on streptococcal disease rates and the carrier state. *New Engl. J. Med.* **249**, 1–9.
39. Percival, A., Armstrong, E.C., and Turner, G.C. (1969) Increased incidence of tetracycline-resistant pneumococci in Liverpool in 1968. *Lancet* i, 998–1000.
40. Karney, W.W., Pedersen, A.H.B., Nelson, M., Adams, H., Pfeiffer, R.T., and Holmes, K.K. (1977) Spectinomycin versus tetracycline for the treatment of gonorrhoea. *New Engl. J. Med.* **296**, 889–94.
41. Brumfitt, W., and Percival, A. (1967) Laboratory control of antibiotic therapy in urinary tract infection. *Ann. N.Y. Acad. Sci.* **145**, 329–43.
42. Report on antibiotic sensitivity test trial organized by the bacteriology committee of the association of clinical pathologists. (1965) *J. clin. Path.* **18**, 1–6.
43. Stokes, E.J., and Waterworth, P.M. Antibiotic sensitivity tests by diffusion methods. *Assoc. clin. Pathologists Broadsheet* 55 (Revised 1972).
44. Pearson, C.H., and Whitehead, J.E.M. (1974) Antibiotic sensitivity testing: a modification of the Stokes method using a rotary plater. *J. clin. Path.* **27**, 430–431.
45. O'Callaghan, C.H., Morris, A., Kirby, S., and Shingler, A.H. (1972) Novel method for detection of β-lactamases by using a chromogenic cephalosporin substrate. *Antimicrob. Agents Chemother.* **1**, 283–8.
46. Noone, P., Parsons, J.M.C., and Pattison, J.R. (1974) Experience in monitoring gentamicin therapy during treatment of serious Gram-negative sepsis. *Br. Med. J.* **1**, 477–84.
47. Waterworth, P.M. (1977) Which gentamicin assay method is the most practicable? *J. antimicrob. Chemother.* **3**, 1–3.
48. Waterworth, P.M. (1973) Laboratory control. In *Antibiotic and chemotherapy,*

eds. Garrod, L.P., Lambert, H.P., and O'Grady, F. Churchill Livingstone, Edinburgh and London, pp. 490–531.

49. Eilard, T., Beskow, D., Norrby, R., Wåhlén, P., and Alestig, K. (1976) Combined treatment with amphotericin B and flucytosine in severe fungal infections. *J. antimicrob. Chemother.* 2, 239–46

50. Newsom, S.W.B. (1977) Rapid sensitivity tests. *J. antimicrob. Chemother.* 3, 201–3.

51. Abraham, E.P. (1949) In *Antibiotics.* Oxford University Press, pp. 1452–8.

52. Rolinson, G.N. (1977) Subinhibitory concentrations of antibiotics. *J. antimicrob. Chemother.* 3, 111–13.

53. Greenwood, D. (1977) In defence of turbidimetry. *J. antimicrob. Chemother.* 3, 286–7.

54. Chabbert, Y.A. (1970) Detection of methicillin and cephalothin resistant staphylococci. In *The control of chemotherapy,* ed. Watt, P.J. Livingstone, Edinburgh and London, pp. 17–24.

55. Petersdorf, R.G., and Sherris, J.C. (1965) Methods and significance of *in vitro* testing of bacterial sensitivity to drugs. *Am. J. Med.* 39, 766–79.

56. Bauer, A.W. (1966) The correlation of sulphonamide disc sensitivity testing with the outcome of therapy in patients with urinary tract infection. *Chemotherapia* 10, 152–60.

57. Percival, A., and Cohen, S.L. (1967) The treatment of peritoneal infections in patients on peritoneal dialysis. *Postgrad. med. J.* 43, Suppl., 160–5.

58. Lowbury, E.J.L., Lilley, H.A., and Kidson, A. (1971) 'Methicillin-resistant' *Staphylococcus aureus:* reassessment by controlled trial in burns unit. *Br. med. J.* 1, 1054–6.

59. Brumfitt, W., and Percival, A. (1971) Antibiotic combinations. *Lancet* i, 387–90.

60. Kerry, D.W., Hamilton-Miller, J.M.T., and Brumfitt, W. (1975) Trimethoprim and rifampicin: *in vitro* activities separately and in combination. *J. antimicrob. Chemother.* 1, 417–27.

61. Neu, H.C. (1977) Mecillinam-an amidino penicillin which acts synergistically with other β-lactam compounds. *J. antimicrob. Chemother.* 3, Suppl. B. 43–52.

Discussion

The discussion on Dr. Percival's paper was held together with a discussion on Dr. Hamilton-Miller's paper. See page 43.

3

Use of laboratory tests in predicting the therapeutic efficacy of antimicrobial compounds

J.M.T. HAMILTON-MILLER

Introduction

Drug companies are compelled to perform large numbers of laboratory tests on each new drug they produce, in order to satisfy the licensing authorities that the drug is a safe and effective one. The tests performed seem to fall into two main groups—firstly, those which seek merely to catalogue the properties of the drug, and secondly, those upon which it is intended that a prediction may be based as to possible clinical applications of the drug. The borderline between these two groups is often very difficult to discern.

Attention will be paid in this paper to tests in the second group: first, the purely *in vitro* ones, such as minimum inhibitory concentration (MIC) determination, protein binding, resistance studies, and work on

31

drug combinations, then those carried out *in vivo*, such as pharmaco-kinetics in man and animals, protection tests, and toxicity studies, and finally, clinical trials will be briefly assessed.

In vitro studies

MIC

Until recently, paramount importance has been attached to this measurement, so much so that it was in danger of its value being over-emphasized. Recent discussions, however, have shown some of its limitations [1, 2]. I wish to suggest that the concept of MIC has only a strictly limited clinical relevance.

More than most microbiological measurements, results of MIC determinations are subject to distortion by error on the part of the experimenter. Some of the possible errors are as follows:

i. Bacterial strains can be selected in such a way that virtually any result can be obtained. To avoid bias, strains should be randomly taken from recent clinical separate isolates, and flora from several centres should be examined.

ii. The type of medium and the inoculum size should be standardized and ideally, a single universal defined medium should be used.

iii. The way in which the end-point is read should be described.

iv. An appropriate reference compound should be tested in parallel.

v. Results must be summarized in a way that is both mathematically acceptable and intelligible to other microbiologists [3]. If the strains tested do not constitute a normally distributed population, it is inappropriate to calculate mean, mode, median, etc.

Much stress is often laid on the importance of differentiating between inhibitory (MIC) and bactericidal (MBC) concentrations. This is a situation (like serum binding) where, although a definite answer is found *in vitro*, generally speaking *in vivo* application is minimal. Drugs like sulphonamides, tetracyclines, and chloramphenicol, all of which are only 'bacteriostatic' *in vitro*, are very effective therapeutical-ly in the normal patient. This is even the case in urinary tract infection, where many of the body's natural defence mechanisms, such as antibody, serum factors, and phagocytosis, are absent. 'Bactericidal' drugs perform better only in some infections with special charac-teristics like subacute bacterial endocarditis, and in compromised patients.

The use of doubling dilutions means that there will inevitably be a large margin of error, even if the end-point can be read precisely. In the tube test, it is worth pointing out that bacterial growth of up to 10^7 organisms/ml will appear non-turbid, and therefore be scored as 'no growth'. Use of a plate method avoids this type of error.

Conditions in the body can vary a great deal—for instance, in terms of pH, oxygen tension, and osmolality; laboratory tests have not always been carried out to show how varying these parameters affects the MIC.

Another important criticism is that MIC determinations are 'single-shot' experiments, where bacteria are in contact with the same concentration of drug for 18 hours. This should be compared with the situation *in vivo*, where the drug concentration may wax and wane several times over this period.

It is now becoming clear that antibiotics can have a substantial effect, morphologically and on growth rate, at concentrations well below the conventionally determined MIC [4]. The relevance of this to the clinical situation is not clear, and it is important that these drugs continue to be used at recommended, as opposed to homeopathic, dosages. However, the fact is that recommended doses very often bear no relation to MIC.

For instance, MIC of cephaloridine for *Staphylococcus aureus* may be one-tenth to one-hundredth that of cephalexin, yet dosage of these antibiotics for soft-tissue infection by this species would probably be the same for both antibiotics—500 mg three or four times daily. One is bound to conclude that there is often little relationship between MIC and clinical performance. There are of course exceptions, as in the case of gentamicin, where Noone *et al.* [5] have shown that better clinical results are obtained by maintaining (intermittently) definitely inhibitory levels.

Complications are introduced when the drug being considered is metabolized *in vivo*. In some cases—such as talampicillin, chloramphenicol palmitate, and methenamine—the substance taken by the patient is a biologically inactive pro-drug. During its passage through the body the pro-drug is converted into the active substance. This process may take varying lengths of time to occur in different subjects, and may indeed be only partial, as in the case of the formation of formaldehyde from methenamine [6]. Often, sophisticated assay methods are necessary to detect pro-drug in the presence of active substance, as in the case of hetacillin [7], or formaldehyde in the presence of methenamine [8]. On the other hand, many antimicrobial agents are metabolized *in vivo* either into a less active form (e.g. cephalothin is converted into desacetylcephalothin) or into inactive substances (e.g. acetylated sulphonamides). The degree of metabolism may vary widely among individuals (e.g. slow and rapid inactivators of isoniazid). A new problem arises when metabolites have an activity which is qualitatively different from that of the original compound.

It is known that several antimicrobial compounds, notably sulphonamides, trimethoprim, and flucytosine, require special media devoid of specific antagonists to show their full activity *in vitro*. *In vivo* it is by no means certain, especially if a pathological process is going on, that some antagonists will be absent. For example, pus may contain free pyrimidines derived from lysed leucocytes [9]; under such conditions trimethoprim will not be as active as would be expected from MIC.

Even if a drug is highly active *in vitro* this is by no means a sure indication that it will be effective therapeutically. Thus, *Salmonella typhi* is highly sensitive *in vitro* to several antibiotics—benzyl-penicillin, streptomycin, polymyxin B, tetracyclines, oxolinic acid, and chloramphenicol for instance [10]—but of these only the latter is active clinically. While it has been shown in serious infections that 'appropriate' antibiotic therapy gives better results than does 'inappropriate' treatment [11], it is not clear that in urinary-tract infections, for instance, treatment using an antibiotic to which a pathogen is 'resistant' would necessarily fail. For ethical reasons such a trial could not, of course, be performed, but, as Bell [12] points out, there is no reason to suppose that all laboratories' results are accurate and relevant. Results of treating infection in general practice if drugs are correctly given are usually excellent. Recourse to sensitivity testing is unnecessary in many cases, e.g. β-haemolytic streptococci, because resistance to penicillin G is unknown.

Protein binding

A great deal of attention is paid in some circles to this phenomenon. It is an undoubted fact that different antibiotics are bound, reversibly, to varying extents to serum proteins, and that the bound fraction is microbiologically inert. Modern techniques allow considerable accuracy in the measurement of such binding. However, it is far from clear how knowledge of the degree of protein binding helps one to predict the likely therapeutic efficacy of an antibiotic. There are several drugs which are very highly bound to human serum protein—for example, fusidic acid and flucloxacillin; conversely, other antibiotics, such as cephalexin and erythromycin, are serum-bound only slightly. These facts cannot be used to predict that cephalexin will be a 'better' or 'worse' drug than flucloxacillin.

Thus, the degree of serum binding of an antibiotic seems to have little relevance to its ultimate clinical performance. A possible exception is in septicaemia, where the concentration of free drug should exceed the estimated MIC.

Resistance studies

A commonly used approach to this problem is to make resistant mutants in the laboratory by 'training' (subculturing in gradually increasing amounts of drug), or by the use of mutagenic agents. This process usually presents little difficulty. However, there is a problem in deciding what the applicability of such results is to the clinical situation. It may be relatively easy to obtain, in the laboratory, mutants which do not occur naturally or are found with extreme rarity. Examples are penicillin-resistant haemolytic streptococci and polyene-resistant yeasts. Hence, a study of naturally-occurring resistant variants is essential. The danger of resistance arising can only be measured by observing what happens when a drug is introduced into practice for a particular indication. It is interesting to note in this respect that experienced workers in the field are divided over whether introducing trimethoprim alone, or rifampicin in combination with another drug for the treatment of non-tuberculous infections, will cause a rapid increase in resistance acquisition to the respective drugs. This situation graphically illustrates the difficulties in making predictions, especially before the agent has been used clinically. It is perhaps worth pointing out that no antimicrobial agent has had to be withdrawn solely because of resistance problems.

Another facet is the existence of resistance mediated by R-factors. Several considerations apply here: how common is the specific R-factor in the community? What is the likelihood of another, incompatible R-factor being present? How effectively does transfer to pathogens occur? What is the spontaneous loss rate of the plasmid? Outbreaks of this type of resistance have in the past tended to be sporadic, self-limiting, and strictly confined to a single geographic location (such as one ward in a hospital). However, there are exceptions to this—notably the recent outbreak of typhoid caused by chloramphenicol-resistant *Salm. typhi* in Mexico and S.E. Asia.

Finally, it must be appreciated that traditionally accepted patterns of cross-resistance now no longer necessarily apply. There are many exceptions, for example, minocycline is active against many tetracycline-resistant strains, and cephalexin inhibits some cephaloridine-resistant strains.

Even when the presence of pre-existing resistant individuals among bacterial populations is found, at relatively high frequencies (such as 10^{-8} for fusidic acid in staphylococci, 10^{-9} in *Escherichia coli* for streptomycin, 10^{-7} to 10^{-8} in Gram-negative rods for rifampicin), this does not necessarily mean that such drug-resistant variants will emerge with great rapidity under therapeutic conditions, making the drug useless. Streptomycin, for instance, was widely used for the treatment of urinary tract infections during the 1950s, and little trouble was experienced with resistance, provided a large dose was used and for a short period of time (up to one week) and the urine kept alkaline. This is despite the fact that there is a high statistical chance of there being at least one resistant *E. coli* in the urinary output of just one day in a patient with significant bacteriuria. Fusidic acid is still very useful for the treatment of staphylococcal infections. It has been shown that it can take as long as one month for resistant tubercle bacilli to emerge during monotherapy of tuberculosis with streptomycin or rifampicin [13].

Combinations

It is now becoming commonplace to read of antimicrobial drugs being tested in combination. To obtain a proper understanding of any interaction, very time-consuming experiments must be done, using many strains of several different species, as it is not possible to predict with any degree of accuracy against which genera (or even species) synergy will be shown. Further, synergy may depend upon a critical ratio between the two compounds. While it is a simple matter to test a certain fixed ratio *in vitro*, it must be remembered that *in vivo* drug ratios will be changing from minute to minute, and will almost certainly be different at any one time in various parts of the body. This is true even with a pair of drugs as well matched in pharmacokinetic terms as trimethoprim and sulphamethoxazole. Thus, the existence of *in vitro* synergy is no guarantee that synergy will also occur under therapeutic conditions. Further, the latter phenomenon is difficult to demonstrate unequivocally (see below).

There seems to be firmer ground in aiming at the suppression of the emergence of resistant mutants as a rationale for combined therapy. While this effect may be easier to demonstrate *in vitro* [14], it has been proved in practice only for tuberculosis.

In vivo studies

Pharmacokinetics

This subject has now developed into a science in its own right, and there is a distressing frequency for papers and textbooks to become more and more complex and less and less applicable to the therapeutic situation. As early studies on new drugs are invariably carried out in animals, possible differences between results obtained in animals and in man must be considered first.

The fate of a drug in the body is governed by four main factors:

i. Absorption: only if a drug is given by the intravenous route can it safely be assumed that all is absorbed into the circulation. It is often the case that a drug absorbed orally by animals will also be absorbed by man, but there are notable exceptions, e.g. tetracycline in rabbits. Whether compounds not absorbed by the oral route by animals are also not absorbed by man does not seem to be known; presumably there are many thousands of compounds which, having failed to be absorbed by animals, have never been tested in man.

ii. Metabolism: many drugs are metabolized *in vivo*. Both the nature and the extent of such metabolism are known to differ widely between animal species (for cephalosporins see [15, 16] and for trimethoprim see [17]).

iii. Distribution: in general animal tissues closely resemble, in physico-chemical terms, human tissue. Hence the distribution patterns of drugs in experimental animals and in man will tend to be broadly similar. Anatomical differences must, however, be borne in mind — such as the facts that rats have no gall bladder and rabbits have a large appendix. Passage of substances across the placenta is known to vary widely even amongst mammalian species.

iv. Excretion: there may be considerable differences in the half-lives of antibiotics in different animals. Examples for trimethoprin and sulphamethoxazole are given in Table 1 (see also [18, 19, 20]).

Thus, it is clear that not much detailed quantitative pharmacokinetic information applicable to man can be deduced from results of animal experiments.

Table 1. Variations in half-life of components of co-trimoxazole according to species.

Species	Half-life (hours)		Reference
	Trimethoprim	Sulphamethoxazole	
Rhesus monkey	1	3	18
Mouse	1	6	19
Man	10–12	10–12	20

Human volunteer studies give much more reliable information. Here again care must be taken before extrapolating directly to the patient situation. Absorption of drugs, by the oral route as well as parenterally, is subject to a wide subject-to-subject variation. The standard deviation may be in the order of $\pm 25\%$ of the mean. What this implies in practical terms is that if a mean level of 10 μg/ml is predictable at a certain time after administration of a drug, the actual values observed will range from 5 to 15 μg/ml in 95% of the observations. Absorption is known to be more erratic in bed-ridden patients than in healthy, ambulant volunteers [21], so this range will be wider in the subject requiring antimicrobial therapy. Bearing in mind that an MIC determined by the doubling dilution technique is subject to an inherent error of virtually $\pm$half its absolute value, the difficulties involved in trying to assess what dose to give in order to obtain a blood level of twice the MIC are obvious.

Another point that is often overlooked is that hospitalized patients are statistically likely to be receiving drugs other than antibiotics [22], which may well have an effect upon the pharmacokinetics of the antibiotic. An example would be a patient on an antacid containing $Al(OH)_3$ who is prescribed tetracycline; multivalent cations chelate with tetracyclines and inhibit absorption.

When tissue perfusion is impaired, as in shock, im drugs may not be absorbed efficiently, and iv treatment becomes necessary.

Volunteer studies are also liable to error if the possible effects of the sex of the subject [23] and the site of the injection [24] are not allowed for. At least one study has shown how a change in the physiological state of the subject may drastically alter the handling of the antibiotic [25].

Clearly, more pharmacokinetic studies are needed in patients. However, this may give rise to ethical problems, especially in those groups where new studies are urgently needed, namely in patients at extremes of age. It is known that both the very young and very old do not handle antibiotics in the same way as do other subjects. For instance, kanamycin and ampicillin (both given im) have considerably prolonged half-lives in premature infants [26]; absorption of ampicillin orally is very poor in neonates, but that of propicillin is better than in more mature infants [27]. Simon *et al.* [28] have shown that cefazolin, cephradine, and sulfisomidine were more slowly excreted and penetrated tissues less well in older subjects.

It must also be remembered that there is as yet no proper assay for tissue levels of antibiotics [29]. Most infections involve the tissues rather than the bloodstream, so monitoring is based chiefly upon guesswork [30]. There is also very little work on most antibiotics as to whether a better clinical effect is obtained by attempting to maintain an inhibitory concentration throughout the course of treatment, as opposed to allowing the drug concentration to fall below the MIC during some period ('continuous' vs. 'intermittent' hypotheses).

Infection models

More attention is now being paid to the whole concept of the relevance of animal protection tests. A widely used model (ip challenge with or without mucin) seems to bear little resemblance to any naturally occurring human infection (except, perhaps, peritonitis). As zoonoses are the exception rather than the rule, it is probably inappropriate to use as challenging organism a bacterial strain isolated from a case of human infection, as this will be an unnatural pathogen for the animal 'model'. More sophisticated models, such as pyelonephritis, are too time-consuming to set up in large numbers. It seems most logical that, when seeking an answer to a question concerning human disease, we should choose the most exact animal model possible: not just the cheapest, easiest or the quickest one. It is probably best, in fact, to use several models. It may not be long before a satisfactory computer model is devised.

Mice seem to have a circadian rhythm with respect to susceptibility to infection [31, 32], so ideally it would be necessary to ensure that all infections were initiated at the same time of day or night. Genetic factors (including sex [33]) are also important in determining susceptibility to infection; this factor may not be easy to quantitate.

To ensure that the desired amount of antibiotic is given, it must be injected. This is done even with compounds normally given orally, such as amoxycillin and cephalexin. In animals the parenteral route chosen is often subcutaneous, one not often used in man. Further, in the model, the duration of treatment is often very short, sometimes as little as two days; this may sometimes give rise to serious error, as in a recently established model of infection with an anaerobe [34], where treatment must last several days. Dosage in the model may not be closely related to that used in man, although there are formulae for converting mouse dose data to human terms [35]. Because of differences previously discussed in the handling of drugs (half-life, metabolism, etc.), it is not really a profitable exercise to try to estimate a reasonable dosage schedule for man from animal experiments. Some of the latter have in fact given definitely misleading results e.g. [36].

There are several pathogens for which either no adequate model animal exists, e.g. venereal diseases, or the model is very new, e.g. the armadillo for leprosy.

Clearly work with animal models will continue, but we should also be looking closely at the model itself.

It is especially difficult to predict clinical synergy in man on the basis of animal experiments. In fact, it may be very hard to prove this type of synergy even by clinical trial. There is evidence that synergy of therapeutic value occurs with co-trimoxazole in gonorrhoea, malaria, toxoplasmosis, and possibly in brucellosis as well; benzylpenicillin and streptomycin undoubtedly act synergistically in subacute bacterial endocarditis due to *Strept. faecalis*, as do carbenicillin and an aminoglycoside in cancer patients [37]. The work of Klastersky, Cappel, and Daneau [38] suggests that the best *in vitro* parameter for predicting synergy is the antibacterial titre of the blood.

Toxicity testing

The introduction of more stringent regulations on the possible toxicity of new and existing drugs raises the whole question of the validity of toxicity testing as at present carried out. This is a very complicated subject with many facets; those interested in the wider aspects of testing for carcinogenicity are referred to recent reviews, two general [39, 40], two more mathematical [35, 41]. A widely used screening method is that devised by Ames, which detects mutagenic activity [42]. It is axiomatic on this rationale that mutagenic equates with carcinogenic; any new compound showing this type of activity is automatically disbarred from use in man. The most acceptable animal model for carcinogenicity is the mouse liver test [43].

As pointed out previously, drugs may be handled in different ways in animals and man. This means that animal tissues will possibly be exposed to very different profiles of time vs. concentration than would occur in man, especially bearing in mind the continual, high-level dosages used. This type of dosage is, however, necessary for statistical purposes, as each mouse may represent 10^6 humans [41].

Species differences, in terms of both susceptibility and the nature of the target site, are of great importance. An especially relevant example is that of thalidomide; it is extremely tragic that man happens to be one of the species most sensitive to the teratogenic effects of this compound. Man is 60 times more sensitive than the mouse, 100 times more than the rat, 200 times more than the dog, and some 700 times more than the hamster [39].

Some of the implications which arise from results of screening antimicrobial compounds for mutagenicity are of considerable interest. For example, nitro compounds are a very versatile group of antimicrobial agents [44], which are useful in many infections, including such widespread scourges as schistosomiasis. Nitrofurantoin and metronidazole are the most familiar members of this group. Studies with these compounds, carried out some time after their clinical value had been firmly established, have shown them to be mutagenic (and, therefore, carcinogenic). As this property seems to be an attribute of the $-NO_2$ moiety (which is also essential for antimicrobial activity), it seems unlikely that any further of this type of compound will be produced, and it is not impossible that existing ones will have to be withdrawn, or their use strictly limited [45]. Griseofulvin, the antifungal agent, is also mutagenic. The question to be asked in connection with these compounds is: will use of them do more harm than would be done by not using them?

Clinical trials

Even well-controlled clinical trials in man cannot provide all the required answers. For instance, they have failed to establish rational dosage schedules: sulphadiazine, for instance, is still prescribed on a 6-hourly basis, although it has a half-life of 10 hours [46]. A decrease in dosage or an increased interval between doses might well have a beneficial effect, especially for the treatment of urinary tract infection, in terms of patient acceptability, cost, incidence of side-effects, and the general effect on microbial ecology.

Ethical constraints clearly forbid the use of 'marginal therapy', which is the only way to establish minimal effective doses. Similarly, for a drug to be pronounced 'safe in pregnancy' may take years to establish, by the laborious means of careful retrospective analysis of those patients known to have taken the drug during pregnancy, and are available for follow-up over a period of years.

Finally, it must be remembered that the best drug ever invented will not work if it is not taken. Patient compliance is a very complex subject about which little is understood, and until recently hardly any notice was taken of it. It should now be considered mandatory for any comparative trial of antimicrobial agents to have built-in checks on compliance.

Summary

It must be concluded that *in vitro* and even *in vivo* studies fail to give us an adequate means of predicting clinical efficiency of antibiotics. Most antimicrobial agents in current use are excellent and in order to show a difference 'difficult' patient groups have to be used [47]. Perhaps the two biggest obstacles standing in our way are firstly, lack of knowledge of tissue levels and secondly, the inappropriateness of currently used animal models [48].

As Alexander Pope put it 'The proper study of mankind is man'.

References

1. Selwyn S. (1976) Unrealistic nature of the 'MIC'. *J. antimicrob. Chemoth.* 2, 221–2.
2. Greenwood, D. (1976) Unrealistic nature of the 'MIC'. *J. antimicrob. Chemoth.* 2, 312–13.
3. Phillips, I., King, A., Warren, C., and Watts, B. (1976) The activity of penicillin and eight cephalosporins on *Neisseria gonorrhoeae*. *J. antimicrob. Chemoth.* 2, 31–9.
4. Lorian, V., and Atkinson, B. (1976) Effects of subinhibitory concentrations of antibiotics on cross walls of cocci. *Antimicrob. Ag. Chemoth.* 9, 1043–55.
5. Noone, P., Parsons, T.M.C., Pattison, J.R., Slack, R.C.B., Garfield-Davies, D., and Hughes, K. (1974). Experience in monitoring gentamicin therapy during treatment of serious Gram-negative sepsis. *Br. med. J.* 1, 477–81.
6. Hamilton-Miller, J.M.T., and Brumfitt, W., (1977) Methenamine and its salts as urinary tract antiseptics: variables affecting the antibacterial activity of formaldehyde, mandelic acid and hippuric acid. *Invest. Urol.* 14, 287–92.
7. Smith, J.T., and Hamilton-Miller, J.M.T. (1970) Hetacillin: a chemical and biological comparison with ampicillin. *Chemotherapy* 15, 366–78.
8. Chen, T.-M., and Chavetz, L. (1972) Selective determination of free urinary formaldehyde after oral dosage with methenamine mandelate. *Invest. Urol.* 10, 212–14.
9. Lacey, R.W., (1977) Personal communication.
10. Sanford, J.P., Linh, N.N., Kutscher, E., Arnold, K., and Gould, K. (1976) Oxolinic acid in the treatment of typhoid fever due to chloramphenicol-resistant strains of *Salmonella typhi. Antimicrob. Ag. Chemoth.* 9, 387–92.
11. McCabe, W.R. (1975) Antibiotics and endotoxic shock. *Bull. New York Acad. Med.* (Second Series) 51, 1084–95.

12. Bell, S. (1976) The relevance of bacteriology tests to the clinical use of antibiotics in domiciliary practice. *J. antimicrob. Chemoth.* **2**, 110–11.
13. Annotation. Rifampicin: for tuberculosis only? *Lancet* **i**, 290–1, 1976.
14. Kerry, D.W., Hamilton-Miller, J.M.T., and Brumfitt, W. (1975) Trimethoprim and rifampicin: *in vitro* activities separately and in combination. *J. antimicrob. Chemoth.* **1**, 417–27.
15. O'Callaghan, C.H., and Muggleton, P.W. (1963) The formation of metabolites from cephalosporin compounds. *Biochem. J.* **89**, 304–8.
16. Cabana, B.E., van Harken, D.R., and Hottendorf, G.H. (1976) Comparative pharmacokinetics and metabolism of cephapirin in laboratory animals and humans. *Antimicrob. Ag. Chemoth.* **10**, 307–17.
17. Sigel, C.W., Grace, M.E., and Nichol. C.A. (1973) Metabolism of trimethoprim in man and measurement of a new metabolite: a new fluorescence assay. *J. inf. Dis.* **128**, S580–3.
18. Craig, W.A., and Kunin, C.M. (1973) Distribution of trimethoprim-sulfamethoxazole in tissues of Rhesus monkeys. *J. inf. Dis.* **128**, S575–9.
19. Böhni, E. (1969) Chemotherapeutic activity of the combination of trimethoprim and sulphamethoxazole in infections of mice. *Postgrad. med. J.* **45**, S18–21.
20. Kaplan, S.A., Weinfeld, R.E., Abruzzo, C.W., McFaden, K., Jack, M.L., and Weissman, L. (1973) Pharmacokinetic profile of trimethoprim-sulfamethoxazole in man. *J. inf. Dis.* **128**, S547–5.
21. Kunst, M.W., and Mattie, H. (1975) Absorption of pivampicillin in postoperative patients. *Antimicrob. Ag. Chemoth.* **8**, 11–14.
22. May, F.E., Stewart, R.B., and Cluff, L.E. (1974) Drug use in hospitals: evaluation of determinants. *Clin. Pharmacol. Therap.* **16**, 834–45.
23. Vukovich, R.A., Brannick, L.J., Sugerman, A.A., and Neiss, E.S. (1975) Sex differences in the intramuscular absorption and bioavailability of cephradine. *Clin. Pharmacol. Therap.* **18**, 215–20.
24. Reeves, D.S., Bywater, M.J., and Wise, R. (1974) Availability of three antibiotics after intramuscular injection into thigh and buttock. *Lancet* **ii**, 1421–2.
25. Nightingale, C.H., Bassaris, H., Tilton, R., and Quintiliani,R. (1975) Changes in pharmacokinetics of cefazolin due to stress. *J. Pharm. Sci.* **64**, 712–14.
26. Michel, M.F., Sorgedrager, N., Driessen, O., Hermans, J., and Kerrebijn, K.F. (1977) Pharmacokinetic study of ampicillin and kanamycin in newborn infants. In *The rational choice of antibacterial agents* (eds. Mouton, R.P., Brumfitt, W., and Hamilton-Miller, J.M.T.), 55–69. Bohn, Scheltema and Holkema, Utrecht, Netherlands.
27. Marget, W., and Wagner, M. (1967) Orale Anwendung von Propicillin, Ampicillin und Dicloxacillin im Säuglingsalter. *Med. Klin.* **62**, 300–5.
28. Simon, C., Malerczyk, V., Tenschert, B., and Möhlenbeck, F. (1976) Die geriatrische Pharmakologie von Cefazolin, Cefradin und Sulfisomidin. *Arzneim.-Forsch.* **26**, 1377–82.
29. Antibiotic tissue concentration, determination and significance. *Infection* **4**, Suppl. 2 S79–170, 1976.
30. Kunin, C.M. (1974) Blood level measurements and antimicrobial agents. *Clin. Pharmacol. Ther.* **16**, 251–6.
31. Feigin, R.D., San Jose, V.H., Haymond, M.W., and Wyatt, R.G. (1969) Daily periodicity of susceptibility of mice to pneumococcal infection. *Nature, Lond.* **224**, 379–80.
32. Wongwiwat, M., Sukapanit, S., Triyanond, C., and Sawyer, W.D. (1972) Circadian rhythm of the resistance of mice to acute pneumococcal infection. *Infect. Immun.* **5**, 442–8.
33. Harle, E.M.J., Bullen, J.J., and Thomson, D.A. (1975) Influence of oestrogen on experimental pyelonephritis caused by *Escherichia coli. Lancet* **ii**, 283–6.
34. Wilkins, T.D., and Smith, L.D.S. (1974) Chemotherapy of an experimental

Fusobacterium (Sphaerophorus) necrophorum infection in mice. *Antimicrob. Ag. Chemoth.* **5**, 658–62.

35. Mantel, N., and Schneiderman, M.A. (1975) Estimating 'safe' levels, a hazardous undertaking. *Cancer Res.* **35**, 1379–86.
36. Muggleton, P.W., O'Callaghan, C.H., Foord, R.D., Kirby, S.M., and Ryan, D.M. (1969) Laboratory appraisal of cephalexin. *Antimicrob. Ag. Chemoth.* –1968, 353–60.
37. Hamilton-Miller, J.M.T., and Brumfitt, W. (1977) Clinical aspects of *in vitro* antimicrobial synergism. In *The rational choice of antibacterial agents* (eds. Mouton, R.P., Brumfitt, W., and Hamilton-Miller, J.M.T.), 89–100. Bohn, Scheltema and Holkema, Utrecht, Netherlands.
38. Klastersky, J., Cappel, R., and Daneau, D. (1972) Clinical significance of *in vitro* synergism between antibiotics in Gram-negative infections. *Antimicrob. Ag. Chemoth.* **2**, 470–5.
39. Epstein, S.S. (1974) Environmental determinants of human cancer. *Cancer Res.* **34**, 242–35.
40. Matter, B.E. (1976) Problems of testing drugs for potential mutagenicity. *Mutation Res.* **38**, 243–58.
41. Hoel, D.G., Gaylor, D.W., Kirschsten, R.L., Saffiotti, U., and Schneiderman M.A. (1975) Estimation of risks of irreversible, delayed toxicity. *J. Toxicol. Environ. Health* **1**, 133–51.
42. McCann, J., Choi, E., Yamasaki, E., and Ames, B.N. (1975) Detection of carcinogens as mutagens in the *Salmonella*/microsome test: assay of 300 chemicals. *Proc. natn. Acad. Sci. U.S.A.* **72**, 5135–9.
43. Tomatis, L., Partensky, C., Montesano, R. (1973) The predictive value of mouse liver tumour induction in carcinogenicity testing—a literature survey. *Int. J. Cancer* **12**, 1–20.
44. Hamilton-Miller, J.M.T., and Brumfitt, W. (1976) The versatility of nitro compounds. *J. antimicrob. Chemoth.* **2**, 5–8.
45. Is Flagyl dangerous? *Medical Letter* **17**, 53–4, 1975.
46. Ohnhaus, E.E., and Spring, P. (1975) Elimination kinetics of sulfadiazine in patients with normal and impaired renal function. *J. Pharmacokin. Biopharm.* **3**, 171–8.
47. Klastersky, J., Swings, G., Vandenborre, L., Weerts, D., and de Maertelaer, V. (1973) Effectiveness of the carbenicillin/cephalothin combination against Gram-negative bacilli. *Am. J. Med. Sci.* **265**, 45–53.
48. O'Grady, F. (1976) Animal models in the assessment of antimicrobial agents: what should we expect of them? In *Chemotherapy* (eds. Williams, J.D. and Geddes A.M.) vol. **2**, 177–81, London.

Discussion

N.B. This discussion also relates to Dr. Percival's paper.

Prof. Asscher: You two have cast rather an air of despair on 'New perspectives in clinical microbiology' and the question I want to put to you and possibly to the other speakers today is regarding the future of clinical microbiology. As a clinician, a point I would like to put to you as microbiologists is whether the control of clinical microbiology ought not to be in the hands of the likes of me. Should the clinicians not run the laboratories rather along the American pattern?

Dr. Percival: I didn't mean my talk to be a counsel of despair. The long established sensitivity tests work, in certain known situations, very well. So they do not need refining. However, there are one or two areas where we know that such refinements are needed. For instance, it has been shown statistically that when gentamicin blood levels are over 8 μg/ml a significant higher cure rate of bacteraemia is found than when levels were below that figure. So here is an area where some degree of laboratory refinement is justified by better results.

Prof. Asscher: So you do not see a future for an infectious disease physician in the laboratory?

Dr. Percival: No. In my view the present system is satisfactory. You can equally argue that it is better that the medical microbiologist makes the link between the laboratory and the patient.

Dr. Willis: Dr. Hamilton-Miller, I would like to clarify your last remarks about the carcinogenicity of some of these compounds. Do you believe that these compounds you refer to are in fact, carcinogenic or are you saying that the FDA believes that, or are you saying that the FDA *and* the Committee on Safety of Medicines in this country believe that? It wasn't clear what you were saying.

Dr. Hamilton-Miller: I personally am not in a position to judge whether a compound is carcinogenic or not. However, on the basis of some expert opinion nitro compounds are *said* to be carcinogenic. Under the Delaney Amendment the FDA have to say that such compounds are not suitable for human use.

Dr. Willis: I would just like to make the point that the FDA is an American body and we are working in the United Kingdom. If we did what the FDA told us, we would be in all sorts of deep trouble. The FDA now recommends (for example) that vaginal trichomoniasis should be treated by douching with vinegar. The Committee on Safety of Medicines in this country license metronidazole with all this evidence before them.

Dr. Percival: The FDA also allows co-trimoxazole only to be used for chronic urinary tract infections at the moment, and they do not allow Fucidin to be used at all.

Dr. Wallace: I am glad Dr. Percival still has faith in laboratory methods. Personally, I am beginning to lose faith in them, even fundamental ones like sensitivity tests. A particular case in point is whether to use a 2-μg and/or a 10-μg ampicillin disc. What is your opinion on this question?

Dr. Percival: It depends what you are testing for. A 2-μg disc is applicable only to Gram-positive organisms, for which ampicillin is very rarely indicated clinically.

Dr. Wallace: It seems to me that a 10-μg disc is too high compared with the levels obtained in the body after the usual dose of ampicillin.

Dr. Percival: I am not sure that I would agree with you on this. A 500 mg dose of ampicillin orally given 6-hourly will often give relief from chronic bronchitis. The late Prof. Robert May reported that 1 gm ampicillin 6-hourly could keep patients free of *H. influenzae* for several months. Some laboratory tests appear to be designed specifically to reduce one's confidence in regimes of known clinical efficiency! Our object should be to devise tests, the results of which mimic clinical results.

Dr. Wallace: What controls would you recommend?

Dr. Percival: I do not believe that one can compare a zone obtained with say, *Strept. faecalis* with that obtained with the Oxford staphylococcus. This practice seems to me illogical. Correlation of zone size with clinical response results from properly carried out clinical trials.

Prof. Brumfitt: Laboratory techniques show that sulphonamides cannot cure urinary tract infections if the classical number of bacteria found in urinary infection is used as an inoculum. However, it is well known that sulphonamides do work in urinary tract infections if the organism is sensitive using an inoculum of 10^3 of the infecting organisms / ml.

Dr. Percival: This is a very good example of where sensitivity testing does not appear to give the correct result. In the case of urinary tract infections there is also the wash-out effect to be taken into consideration.

Prof. O'Grady: I agree that this is a classic example of the fact that the conditions in which the MIC is done are nothing like the conditions in which the drug operates in the patient: if you test sulphonamides in the bladder model they work extremely well, but you have to wait long enough to wash out the organisms that have a big enough folate pool to survive initial contact with sulphonamide until it starts to work. However, as Professor Brumfitt has indicated, patients don't get treated with one dose overnight in a static situation, but by multiple doses in a highly dynamic situation.

Dr. Percival: Can I add one word. I think microbiologists can cause harm. One part of controlling antibiotic policy is by controlling the sensitivity tests that you send out. One authority tells us only to report as 'co-trimoxazole-sensitive' organisms which are sensitive to sulphonamides. Now I think that this is very bad because if you do this the clinicians will cease to have any confidence in your reports. If you want to have a hospital policy where they agree only to use co-trimoxazole under those conditions that's one thing but you shouldn't manipulate the sensitivity reports and tell a lie to try and impose a policy. I won't do that in my hospital until someone shows me that co-trimoxazole clinically has been associated with an increase in trimethoprim-resistant strains and so far all the figures I have in community medicine show the reverse.

Prof. O'Grady: My worry about that is that there is such a word as co-trimoxazole.

Dr. Percival: Well, there is. We can't do anything about it.

Prof. Brumfitt: Could I make another point. The title of the talk is how to control chemotherapy in the laboratory and there has been a lot of discussion about aminoglycosides. Dr. Sabath, whom I regard as a very careful worker, feels that estimations on the 2nd, 3rd and 4th day of the trough level is enough for control of therapeutic efficacy and avoiding toxicity. Provided you are not getting accumulation you do not get 8th-nerve damage.

Dr. Percival: I am very pleased to hear that. In 1946 they were arguing about whether a constant or fluctuating level of antibiotic was preferable. Now, after thirty years we know about the traditional fluctuating levels and that they work. Secondly, if tissue levels have any significance they are likely to be lower than peak serum levels and they are likely to have a much flatter curve than the traditional blood level.

Dr. Hamilton-Miller: There have been reports of the use of constant infusion pumps. The clinicians reported there were better results when a constant level of say 10 μg/ml was maintained rather than when the drug was given by bolus intravenous or intramuscular injection. Thus, there is some evidence at least for the aminoglycosides that better clinical results are achieved by maintaining a constant level in the blood.

Dr. Williamson: I would like to correct one statement that Dr. Hamilton-Miller made. It was in the late 1940s that it was realized that aminoglycosides were much less active anaerobically than aerobically.

Dr. Hamilton-Miller: Yes, I agree but of course this was only for streptomycin and for a small number of strains. Our study involved several aminoglycosides and a considerable number of strains. The question of the decreased activity of some of the newer aminoglycosides under anaerobic conditions has been investigated by us (Reynolds, Hamilton-Miller and Brumfitt (1976) *Lancet*).

4

Metronidazole in the prevention and treatment of bacteroides infections in surgical patients

A.T. WILLIS

Abstract

Clinical trials were carried out in order to determine the value of metronidazole in preventing the development of anaerobic infections after surgery. Following a successful controlled trial of hysterectomy patients, among whom the prophylactic use of oral metronidazole resulted in a reduction of the anaerobic sepsis rate from 23% to nil, further trials were carried out with patients having urgent appendicectomy and those having elective colonic surgery. These studies were conducted as double-blind trials in which metronidazole was compared with a placebo; patients were randomly allocated to the two 'drug' groups.

Among appendicectomy patients, anaerobic infection did not develop in any of 49 patients who received prophylactic metronidazole, but bacteriologically confirmed clinical anaerobic infections developed in nine (19%) of 46 control patients. Since completion of the trial over 800 appendicectomies have been performed under metronidazole cover, only one of which developed an anaerobic infection.

Among colonic surgery patients, anaerobic infections did not develop in any of 27 patients who received prophylactic metronidazole, but bacteriologically confirmed clinical anaerobic infections developed in 11 (58%) of 19 control patients. Since completion of the trial over 70 colonic operations have been performed under metronidazole cover, none of which was complicated by anaerobic sepsis.

Metronidazole is regarded as the drug of choice for the prevention of post-surgical anaerobic sepsis and for the treatment of those non-clostridial anaerobic infections that require antimicrobial therapy.

Introduction

Metronidazole ('Flagyl') has been used for many years to treat trichomonal and giardial infections. As the result of a chance observation by Shinn [1] that the drug was also highly effective in the treatment of Vincent's stomatitis, metronidazole is now generally accepted as the drug of choice in this condition.

Since Vincent's stomatitis is caused by Gram-negative anaerobic microorganisms, the activity of metronidazole against a wide variety of clinically important anaerobes has been determined [2-10]. It is now clear that metronidazole has a universally bactericidal effect on anaerobic organisms, that aerobic and facultatively anaerobic bacteria are universally resistant to it, and that the *in-vitro* minimum inhibitory and minimum bactericidal concentrations of the drug are equivalent. Extensive experience in patients treated with metronidazole for trichomonal infection has shown that the drug is virtually non-toxic and free from side-effects in man, and that blood serum levels are readily obtained that are far in excess of that theoretically required for successful antibacterial therapy [11-13].

Recently there has been an increasing awareness of the importance of non-sporing anaerobes as the major cause of sepsis after surgery of the gastrointestinal tract and female genital tract [14-16]. This matter has been highlighted in relation to appendicitis by Leigh *et al.* [17], who recovered *Bacteroides fragilis* from 90% of wound infections after appendicectomy. Experience at the Luton and Dunstable Hospital leaves no room for doubt that most infections that develop after intestinal surgery (especially of the large bowel) and major gynaecological surgery (especially hysterectomy) are caused by non-sporing anaerobes. These organisms, especially the *Bacteroides*, are normal inhabitants of the vagina and of the gastrointestinal tract, whence they invade traumatized tissues, thus causing endogenous infections.

The present report reviews experience with metronidazole at the Luton and Dunstable Hospital, England, where the drug has been extensively used in the prevention and treatment of bacteroides infections in surgical patients.

Three different categories of surgical patient were studied in controlled trials; these were patients having elective hysterectomy, patients having elective colonic surgery, and those having emergency appendicectomy. In each surgical category one group of patients was given prophylactic metronidazole therapy, aimed at reducing the incidence of postoperative anaerobic infection; a second control group in each category received only placebo. This prophylactic approach was adopted for the following reasons:

1. Metronidazole is therapeutically safe, non-toxic, and virtually without side-effects.

2. Metronidazole is totally inactive against aerobic and facultatively anaerobic bacteria, so that its clinical use can have no directly adverse effect on normal populations of these organisms in the body. Moreover, any reduction of the postoperative infection rate in patients receiving metronidazole may be confidently attributed to a specific reduction in the infection rate due to anaerobes.

3. Initially, it was not possible to justify the use of metronidazole for the empirical treatment of patients severely ill with anaerobic infections, knowing that other well-tried and highly effective drugs, such as clindamycin, are available. However, demonstration of its value in prophylaxis would add weight to the argument for its therapeutic use.

Hysterectomies

The development of pelvic cellulitis or pelvic abscess following hysterectomy is a not uncommon experience, and it is clear that most of these 'vaginal cuff' infections are due to non-sporing anaerobic bacteria derived from the normal vaginal flora [17-20]. Previous studies have shown that the incidence of this post-surgical sepsis may be significantly reduced by the prophylactic use of chloramphenicol [21], of penicillin and streptomycin [22] and of cephaloridine [23].

Method of study

All patients admitted to the gynaecological ward for elective hysterectomy were admitted to the study, provided that there was no recent history of antibiotic or metronidazole therapy and no evidence of existing infection. Alternate patients were given prophylactic metronidazole orally according to one or other of the following schedules: those patients admitted 24 hours before operation were given metronidazole 2 g on admission, then 200 mg 3 times a day postoperatively for 7 days; and those admitted 48 hours before operation were given metronidazole 2 g on admission, then 200 mg 3 times a day to the end of the 7th postoperative day (the drug course was interrupted during the period of preoperative starvation). Full details of the methods employed were published by the Study Group [24, 25].

Frequency of postoperative pelvic infection caused by anaerobes

During their stay in hospital and subsequently in a convalescent home (average 14 days) anaerobic infection did not develop in any of 74 patients who received prophylactic metronidazole. In contrast, bacteriologically confirmed clinical infections due to anaerobic organisms developed in 18 (23%) of 78 control patients (Table 1). Among the 74 patients who received prophylactic metronidazole, one developed an anaerobic pelvic infection 28 days postoperatively (14 days after discharge from hospital).

Nine patients with pelvic infections caused by non-clostridial anaerobes who required antimicrobial therapy were successfully treated with oral metronidazole.

Table 1. Postoperative anaerobic infections among 152 hysterectomy patients

Group	No. of patients postoperatively	
	Not infected	Infected
Metronidazole	73	1 (late)
Controls	60	18

$$\chi^2 = 14.7; \ P < 0.005$$

Rectal administration of metronidazole

During the course of the gynaecological study a number of patients were seen who required urgent gynaecological surgery, and in whom it was considered that preoperative prophylactic or therapeutic metronidazole would have been of value. Administration of metronidazole by the oral route was clearly inappropriate for acute surgical patients. Although it is entirely feasible to administer the drug intravenously, it was regarded as undesirable to use this route in such a study. The obvious alternative was to give the drug rectally, provided acceptable serum levels could be achieved.

In a small pilot study among healthy male volunteers, metronidazole was administered by retention enema and by suppositories. Thirty minutes after administration of 500 mg of metronidazole by retention enema, the mean serum level in volunteers was 4.0 μg/ml (range 3.5 to 4.8 μg/ml). Peak values were reached between ½ and 1 hour after administration. Six hours after medication the mean level was 2.8 μg/ml (range 2.2 to 3.5 μg/ml).

One hour after administration of 1 g of metronidazole by suppository, the mean serum level in volunteers was 2.3 μg/ml (range 1.0 to 4.8 μg/ml). Peak values were generally reached at about the 4th hour, when the mean serum level was 10.5 μg/ml (range 7.6 to 15.6 μg/ml).

Appendicectomies

Acute appendicitis is a common condition that usually requires emergency surgery. The commonest complication of appendicectomy is undoubtedly surgical sepsis, the incidence of which may vary from 4% for normal appendices to 77% for gangrenous or perforated appendices. The average frequency of postoperative infection is probably about 30% [26-29]. Although some of these infections are relatively trivial they often delay discharge from hospital and subsequent return to work, some are serious or even life-threatening. In an effort to reduce the incidence of sepsis after appendicectomy surgeons have used various topical and systemic prophylactic antibacterial agents. Topical prophylactic agents have included ampicillin, polybactrin, and tetracycline. Ampicillin, tetracycline, penicillin, lincomycin, clindamycin, gentamicin, and tobramycin have all been used systemically [17, 28, 30, 34].

Although none of the prophylactic procedures reported is consistently effective, appropriate systemic antibiotics generally reduce the incidence of intra-abdominal sepsis, while appropriate local treatment reduces the incidence of wound infection [28, 31, 33]. Most reports on the chemoprophylaxis of sepsis after appendicectomy have been concerned solely with clinical aspects of infection and have not considered the nature of the infecting agents. This is unfortunate because in this connection the effectiveness of any prophylactic antibiotic clearly depends on its spectrum of antibacterial activity. It is still widely believed that abdominal infections after surgery are usually caused by the *Enterobacteriaceae* and enterococci. As long ago as 1898, however, Veillon and Zuber [35] reported on the common occurrence of non-sporing anaerobes in cases of appendicitis, an observation that was subsequently confirmed and amplified upon by Altemeier [36]. It was also shown by Altemeier [37] that the foul-smelling pus, which is so commonly associated with these infections, is always due to non-sporing anaerobes, and that true *Escherichia coli* pus is odourless.

Method of study

All patients entering the hospital for emergency appendicectomy were admitted to the trial provided that there was no recent history of antibiotic or metronidazole treatment. The study was conducted as a double-blind trial in which metronidazole was compared with a placebo. Patients were randomly allocated to the two groups.

With the preoperative medication 1 g of metronidazole or placebo was given rectally in a 4-g Witepsol suppository. These suppositories consisted of 2 g of Witepsol 35, 1 g of Witepsol 75, and 1 g of metronidazole or placebo. After surgery each patient received one suppository every eight hours until oral feeding began, when metronidazole or placebo was given in tablets—200 mg three times daily to the end of the seventh day. Children under 12 years received small paediatric suppositories which contained 0.5 g of metronidazole or placebo. For full details of methods see [38].

Frequency of post-appendicectomy infection caused by anaerobes

Anaerobic infection did not develop in any of 49 patients who received prophylactic metronidazole, but bacteriologically confirmed clinical anaerobic infection developed in nine (19%) of 46 control patients (Table 2). Clinically all of the infected patients were feverish and ill, and there were copious foul-smelling discharges from their wounds,

Table 2. Postoperative anaerobic infections among 95 appendicectomy patients

Group	No. of patients postoperatively	
	Not infected	Infected
Metronidazole	49	0
Controls	37	9

$$\chi^2 = 8.4; \ P < 0.005$$

usually without evidence of superficial inflammation. Although exploration was not undertaken all of these infections were judged to be deep-seated and to be due to non-sporing anaerobes.

Four of the nine control patients who developed postoperative anaerobic infections were treated with 'watchful expectancy'. The fever generally resolved in five to seven days, and the discharge stopped and healing began soon afterwards. In the other five infected patients the infection was severe enough to warrant antibacterial treatment. Reference to the double-blind trial code showed that none of them was receiving prophylactic metronidazole, and the drug was then given therapeutically according to the prophylactic schedule already outlined. In all cases the temperature settled within 24 hours, with subsequent cessation of discharge and uneventful recovery.

Colonic surgery

Gastrointestinal surgery is associated with a high incidence of postoperative sepsis due to contamination to the field of operation by organisms derived from the intestine. An incidence of serious sepsis in excess of 50% is common following colonic surgery [39-42].

Although the value of preoperative mechanical emptying of the bowel is not disputed, the use of prophylactic antibiotics in the preparation of patients for elective bowel surgery has remained controversial [34, 43-47]. Most studies of antibiotic prophylaxis have been concerned with control of infections due to aerobic bacteria, against which even prolonged courses of systemic antibiotics have frequently proved ineffective. Clearly the rational use of prophylactic antibiotics in colonic surgery requires an understanding of the bacterial flora encountered during surgery and of the sensitivity of the bacteria to various antibiotics.

Method of study

All patients admitted to the Luton and Dunstable Hospital for elective colonic surgery during a 9-month period were admitted to the trial, provided that there was no recent history of antibiotic or metronidazole therapy. The study was a double-blind trial using active and placebo suppositories and tablets. Patients were randomly allocated to the metronidazole and placebo groups.

There were 46 patients studied, 27 of whom received metronidazole and 19 of whom were controls. Most operations were for malignant disease (21 among metronidazole patients and 15 among controls). The remaining 10 patients suffered from diverticular disease (two in each group), Crohn's disease (one in each group), ulcerative colitis (one in each group), and perforation of large bowel (two in metronidazole group). Patients in the two groups were moderately well-matched for sex, age, underlying pathology, operative procedure, and state of bowel at operation.

Before operation all patients were prepared with mechanical evacuation of the bowel. Twenty-four hours preoperatively an oral dose of metronidazole of 1 g or placebo was given, followed by one 200-mg tablet 8-hourly until preoperative starvation; this regimen

53

aimed at achieving early and adequate blood and tissue concentrations. As part of the preoperative medication each patient was given a single intramuscular injection of 80 mg gentamicin, and a Witepsol-base suppository rectally that contained either 1 g of metronidazole or placebo.

At operation, clearly, no uniform technique for colonic surgery was possible. The four surgical teams taking part in the study used a routine preoperative skin preparation. No other antibacterial agents were used during surgery. After operation the surgeons recorded details of operative technique and clinical findings on a form.

After operation patients continued to receive metronidazole or placebo prophylaxis until the end of the seventh postoperative day. With few exceptions each patient received one suppository every eight hours until oral feeding began, when 200-mg tablets of metronidazole or placebo were given three times daily. If suppositories could not be administered rectally, they were administered per colostomy. Two patients with ileostomy who tended to reject suppositories were successfully given metronidazole or placebo via a nasogastric tube as a suspension of the powder (200 mg 8-hourly). Satisfactory blood concentrations of metronidazole (of the order of 2.5 μg/ml after 1 hour) were achieved, although routine aspiration of the stomach was continued at hourly intervals. No other antimicrobial agents were used. Full details of the methods employed have been published [48].

Frequency of postoperative infection caused by anaerobes

Anaerobic infections did not develop in any of 27 patients who received prophylactic metronidazole, but bacteriologically confirmed clinical anaerobic infections developed in 11 (58%) of 19 control patients (Table 3). This remarkable difference in the anaerobic sepsis

Table 3. Postoperative anaerobic infections among 46 colonic surgery patients

Group	No. of patients postoperatively	
	Not infected	Infected
Metronidazole	27	0
Controls	8	11

$$\overline{\chi^2} = 17.8; \ P < 0.0005$$

rate between the two groups of patients is similar to that reported by Goldring *et al.* [44], who used kanamycin and metronidazole for the preoperative 'sterilization' of the gut. All 11 infected patients in the present study were feverish and ill, and there were foul-smelling discharges from their wounds, usually copious and without evidence of superficial inflammation; all of these infections were judged to be deep-seated and due to non-sporing anaerobes. In one patient there was breakdown of the perineal wound, in another abdominal wound dehiscence, and a third patient developed severe *Bacteroides fragilis* bacteraemia. Among the 11 patients who developed postoperative anaerobic infections reference to the double-blind trial code showed that none of them was receiving prophylactic metronidazole, and the drug was then given therapeutically, along the general lines outlined in the prophylactic schedule; gentamicin was sometimes also given. In all cases the temperature settled within 12–24 hours, with subsequent cessation of discharge and uneventful recovery from the infection.

Implications and conclusions

The studies reviewed above have shown that a bactericidal concentration of metronidazole in the blood sustained during and after operation greatly reduces the frequency of postoperative infection. Although the potential of metronidazole in the treatment of anaerobic infections has been recognized for some time [7], its assessment has been delayed by the fact that only an oral preparation has been available. For patients who can take food by mouth oral metronidazole is highly effective in both the prophylaxis and treatment of anaerobic infections [24, 25, 38, 48–51]. Independent studies at Newcastle and Luton (England) have shown that the drug may be administered effectively and safely by the intravenous and rectal routes. Ingham *et al.* [51] described the use of intravenous metronidazole in three patients with otogenic brain abscesses due to bacteroides, and the rectal route was first used in a patient with septic abortion due to *B. fragilis* after a successful trial of this route in healthy volunteers [25]. From the serum metronidazole levels obtained in patients who received active suppositories [38] it is clear that administration of the drug in this form is therapeutically appropriate. Moreover, administration by the rectal route incurred no side-effects, administration was easy for the nursing staff and acceptable to patients, and suppositories could be given to virtually all patients of all ages who could not take anything by mouth—for example, the unconscious patient and those undergoing preoperative starvation or with paralytic ileus.

The absolute inactivity of metronidazole against aerobic bacteria, and its remarkable efficacy in reducing the incidence of post-surgical sepsis clearly implies that most of the infections that complicate appendicectomy and gynaecological and colonic surgery have an anaerobic bacterial aetiology. Confirmation of this was provided by the bacteriological findings among those control patients who developed clinical postoperative infections. Conclusions of this sort cannot be drawn from similar prophylactic studies in which a single broad-spectrum drug, such as a cephalosporin, or mixtures of drugs such as gentamicin and lincomycin have been used. Nor can they be inferred from studies of chemical antiseptics such as povidone-iodine, which are usually unselective, 'total' bactericidal agents. We believe that antimicrobial prophylaxis of endogenously derived anaerobic infections requires the presence of an appropriate drug circulating in the patients' blood at the time of surgery. This requirement cannot be met by the use of antiseptics.

The earlier studies reviewed here of metronidazole treatment used the prophylactic approach in order to determine the possible therapeutic value of the drug. It soon became clear that metronidazole prevented the development of most severe postoperative sepsis. This finding has been substantiated by subsequent experience at the Luton and Dunstable Hospital, where metronidazole prophylaxis is now used routinely in all patients having hysterectomy, appendicectomy and colonic surgery; anaerobic sepsis is never encountered. It is perhaps significant that burst abdomen has not been seen in patients receiving metronidazole prophylaxis, although wound dehiscence was not a rare complication of abdominal surgery prior to introduction of the drug. Despite other elegant and ingenious explanations of its aetiology it seems likely that burst abdomen is commonly a direct result of an aerobic infection.

Although it is beyond our competence to discuss the contemporary philosophy of antibiotic prophylaxis, it is difficult to reconcile its theoretical disadvantages with the practical reality that anaerobic infection is a common and often life-threatening complication of gastrointestinal and female genital tract surgery. In our view, failure to employ thoughtful preventive treatment is as difficult to justify as the use of indiscriminate 'shot-gun' prophylaxis.

The considerable reduction in postoperative morbidity due to metronidazole prophylaxis has not only shortened patients' stay in hospital and thus made available additional beds but has lightened the nursing of patients with serious postoperative sepsis by virtually eliminating it. It is pertinent to note that each of these surgical studies was terminated prematurely because the findings engendered a belief that it is improper to withhold metronidazole prophylaxis from these categories of surgical patients.

The fairly conventional dosage schedules of metronidazole used in these studies were chosen arbitrarily, since the requirement was only to obtain adequate blood metronidazole concentrations, no close attention being paid to the pharmacokinetics of the drug. These schedules were probably more than adequate, and in future it should be possible to reduce both the dosage and the duration of treatment without adversely affecting the protection afforded. Toxic or other untoward effects were never encountered. Although use of the rectal route is regarded as a clinical novelty by some, administration is easy for the nursing staff and acceptable to patients; it is exceedingly uncommon for suppositories to be rejected except by patients in labour.

Since the completion of these studies metronidazole prophylaxis has been used routinely in our hospital for all patients undergoing colonic and gynaecological surgery. This policy of routine prophylaxis would need to be reconsidered if metronidazole resistance was shown to develop *in vivo*; no such acquired resistance has yet been encountered. Moreover, prolonged efforts have failed altogether to induce stable resistance *in vitro* to metronidazole among strains of *B. fragilis* (Ferguson, personal communication). Since aerobic bacteria are all inherently resistant to metronidazole, these organisms do not impose the sorts of constraints upon its prophylactic use that may apply to broad-spectrum drugs such as lincomycin and β-lactam antibiotics.

Because metronidazole is totally inactive against aerobic and facultatively anaerobic bacteria, its prophylactic use can have no direct effect on the incidence of postoperative infection due to these organisms. In each of the three surgical categories of patient studied at Luton there was a low incidence of wound sepsis (about 5%) due exclusively to facultative anaerobes; this sepsis was almost always localized, superficial and mild, without accompanying systemic symptoms, and rarely requiring antimicrobial therapy. Although it is possible that a combination of drugs, such as gentamicin with metronidazole, might have abolished *all* forms of post-surgical sepsis, it is probably neither necessary nor wise to use a broad-spectrum antibiotic against sepsis that is both trivial and uncommon.

In all patients who were infected with anaerobic bacteria the clinical and microbiological response to metronidazole was dramatic. Within 12–24 hours the temperature and pulse rate had usually returned to normal, the patient felt and looked better and there was clear evidence of resolution of any cellulitis. There was a strikingly rapid disappearance of anaerobic bacteria from pathological discharges, which ceased to be purulent and offensive and quickly subsided.

In view of the remarkable systemic activity of metronidazole it is not surprising that the drug is also an effective topical agent. It has been used successfully as a sterile 1% aqueous solution for the irrigation of infected soft-tissue sinuses and abscess cavities, and as a dressing lotion for infected pressure sores, and varicose and diabetic ulcers. In these clinical settings topical metronidazole not only combats anaerobic infection but it has the additional social advantage of abolishing any offensive odour.

Whatever views may be held about the prophylactic as opposed to the therapeutic use of metronidazole, the experience reviewed here adds considerable weight to the proposal that metronidazole should now be regarded as the drug of choice for the prevention of these infections and for the treatment of those non-clostridial anaerobic infections that require antimicrobial therapy.

Future studies may well show that metronidazole has an important place in the conservative management of appendicitis when surgical intervention must be delayed, as may occur, for example, in the submarine service; and Fiddian (personal communication) has suggested that the drug may be a useful prophylactic for military personnel when exposed to the risk of perforating injuries to the gastrointestinal tract in battle.

Acknowledgements

This paper reviews studies carried out over a 4-year period by a Study Group at the Luton and Dunstable Hospital. Reports by the Study Group were first published in the *Lancet*, [24] the *Journal of Antimicrobial Chemotherapy*, [25] and the *British Medical Journal*, [38 45 48] whose Editors I thank for their permission to use that material in this review.

References

1. Shinn, D.S. (1962) Metronidazole in acute ulcerative gingivitis. *Lancet* i, 1191.
2. Davies, A.H., McFadzean, J.A., and Squires, S. (1964) Treatment of Vincent's stomatitis with metronidazole. *Br. med. J.* 1, 1149.
3. Freeman, W.A., McFadzean, J.A., and Whelan, J.P.F. (1968) Activity of metronidazole against experimental tetanus and gas gangrene. *J. app. Bact.* 31, 443–7.
4. McFadzean, J.A., Squires, S.L., and Whelan, J.P.F. (1969) The interactions of metronidazole and micro-organisms. *Medicine Today* 3, 13–14.
5. Prince, H.N., Grunberg, E., Titsworth, E., and DeLorenzo, W.F. (1969) Effects of 1-(2-nitro-1-imidazolyl)-3-methoxy-2-propanol and 2-methyl-5-nitroimidazole-1-ethanol against anaerobic and aerobic bacteria and protozoa. *App. Microbiol.* 18, 728–30.
6. Ueno, K., Ninomiya, K., and Suzuki, S. (1971) Antibacterial activity of metronidazole against anaerobic bacteria. *Chemotherapy, Japan* 19, 111–14.
7. Tally, F.P., Sutter, V.L., and Finegold, S.M. (1972) Metronidazole versus anaerobes. *In vitro* data and initial clinical observations. *California Med.* 117, 22–6.
8. Nastro, L.J., and Finegold, S.M. (1972) Bactericidal activity of five antimicrobial agents against *Bacteroides fragilis*. *J. infec. Dis.* 126, 104–7.
9. Whelan, J.P.F., and Hale, J.H. (1973) Bactericidal activity of metronidazole against *Bacteroides fragilis*. *J. clin. Path.* 26, 393–5.
10. Ingham, H.R., Selkon, J.B., and Hale, J.H. (1975) The antibacterial activity of metronidazole. *J. antimicrob. Chemother.* 1, 355–61.
11. Gray, M.S., Kane, P.O., and Squires, S. (1961) Further observations on metronidazole (Flagyl). *Br. J. vener. Dis.* 37, 278–9.
12. Kane, P.O., McFadzean, J.A., and Squires, S. (1961) Absorption and excretion of metronidazole. II. Studies on primary failures. *Br. J. vener. Dis.* 37, 276–7.
13. McFadzean, J.A. (1969) The absorption, distribution and metabolism of metronidazole. *Medicine Today* 3, 10–12.

14. Chow, A.W., Marshall, J.R., and Guze, L.B. (1975) Anaerobic infections of the female genital tract: prospects and perspectives. *Obstet. Gynec. Survey* **30**, 477–94.
15. Gorbach, S.L., and Bartlett, J.G. (1974) Anaerobic infections. *New Engl. J. Med.* **290**, 1177–84, 1237–45, 1289–94.
16. Willis, A.T., Young, S.E.J., and Ferguson, I.R. (1974) Infections due to non-sporing anaerobes: Some illustrative cases. In *Infection with non-sporing anaerobic bacteria*; Eds. I. Phillips and M. Sussman, pp. 189–201. Churchill Livingstone, London.
17. Hall, W.L., Sobel, A.I., Jones, C.P., and Parker, R.T., (1967) Anaerobic postoperative pelvic infections. *Obstet. Gynec.* **30**, 1–7.
17a. Leigh, D.A., Simmons, K., and Norman, E. (1974) Bacterial flora of the appendix fossa in appendicitis and postoperative wound infection. *J. clin. Path.* **27**, 997–1000.
18. Swenson, R.M., Michaelson, T.C., Daly, M.J., and Spaulding, E.H. (1973) Anaerobic bacterial infections of the female genital tract. *Obstet. Gynec.* **42**, 538–41.
19. Neary, M.P., Allen, J., Okubadejo, O.A., and Payne, D.J.H. (1973) Preoperative vaginal bacteria and postoperative infections in gynaecological patients. *Lancet* **ii**, 1291–4.
20. Craft, I., Ghandi, F., and Hardy, R. (1974) Bacteroides in gynaecological infection. *Lancet* **i**, 677.
21. Goosenberg, J., Emich, J.P., and Schwartz, R.H. (1969) Prophylactic antibiotics in vaginal hysterectomy. *Am. J. Obstet. and Gynec.* **105**, 503–6.
22. Harralson, J.D., Nagell, J.R. van, Roddick, J.W., and Sprague, A.D. (1974) The effect of prophylactic antibiotics on pelvic infection following vaginal hysterectomy. *Am. J. Obstet. Gynec.* **120**, 1046–49.
23. Ledger, W.J., Sweet, R.L., and Headington, J.T. (1973) Prophylactic cephaloridine in the prevention of postoperative pelvic infections in premenopausal women undergoing vaginal hysterectomy. *Am. J. Obstet. Gynec.* **115**, 766–84.
24. Study Group (1974) Metronidazole in the prevention and treatment of *Bacteroides* infections in gynaecological patients. *Lancet* **ii**, 1540–3.
25. Study Group (1975) An evaluation of metronidazole in the prophylaxis and treatment of anaerobic infections in surgical patients. *J. antimicrob. Chemother.* **1**, 393–401.
26. *The Lancet* (1970) Wound infection after appendicectomy. **i**, 930.
27. *The Lancet* (1971) Sepsis after appendicectomy. **ii**, 195.
28. Magarey, C.J., Chant, A.D.B., Rickford, C.R.K., and Magarey, J.R. (1971) Peritoneal drainage and systemic antibiotics after appendicectomy. *Lancet* **ii**, 179–82.
29. Airan, M.C., Levine, H.D., and Sice, J. (1973) Prevention of wound infection. *Lancet* **i**, 1058.
30. Rickett, J.W.S., and Jackson, B.T. (1969) Topical ampicillin in the appendicectomy wound: report of double-blind trial. *Br. med. J.* **4**, 206–7.
31. Longland, C.J., Gray, J.G., Lees, W., and Garrett, J.A.M. (1971) The prevention of infection in appendicectomy wounds. *Br. J. Surg.* **58**, 117–19.
32. Benson, E.A., Brown, G.J.A., and Whittaker, M. (1973) Prevention of wound infection in acute appendicitis. *Lancet* **ii**, 322.
33. Bates, T., Down, R.H.L., Houghton, M.C.V., and Lloyd, G.J. (1974) Topical ampicillin in the prevention of wound infection after appendicetomy. *Br. J. Surg.* **61**, 489–92.
34. Stokes, E.J., Waterworth, P.M., Franks, V., Watson, B., and Clark, C.G. (1974) Short term routine antibiotic prophylaxis in surgery. *Br. J. Surg.* **61**, 739–42.
35. Veillon, M.A., and Zuber (1898) Studies on some strict anaerobic bacteria and their role in pathology. *Archs Méd. exp. Anat. path.* **10**, 517–45.

36. Altemeier, W.A. (1938a) The bacterial flora of acute perforated appendicitis with peritonitis. *Ann. Surg.* **107**, 517–28.
37. Altemeier, W.A. (1938b) The cause of the putrid odor of perforated appendicitis with peritonitis. *Ann. Surg.* **107**, 634–46.
38. Study Group (1976) Metronidazole in prevention and treatment of bacteroides infections after appendicectomy. *Br. med. J.* **1**, 318–21.
39. Everett, M.T., Brogan, T.D., and Nettleton, J. (1969) The place of antibiotics in colonic surgery: A clinical study. *Br. J. Surg.* **56**, 679–84.
40. Jackson, D.W., Pollock, A.V., and Tindal, D.S. (1971) The value of a plastic adhesive drape in the prevention of wound infection. *Br. J. Surg.* **58**, 340–2.
41. Davidson, A.I.G., Smith, G., and Smylie, H.G. (1971) A bacteriological study of the immediate environment of a surgical wound. *Br. J. Surg.* **58**, 326–33.
42. Burton, R.C. (1973) Postoperative wound infection in colonic and rectal surgery. *Br. J. Surg.* **60**, 363–5.
43. Nichols, R.L., Broido, P., Condon, R.E., Gorbach, S.L., and Nyhus, L.M. (1973) Effect of preoperative neomycin–erythromycin intestinal preparation on the incidence of infectious complications following colon surgery. *Ann. Surg.* **178**, 453–62.
44. Goldring, J., Scott, A., McNaught, W., and Gillespie, G. (1975) Prophylactic oral antimicrobial agents in elective colonic surgery. *Lancet* **ii**, 997–1000.
45. Griffiths, D.A., Shorey, B.A., Simpson, R.A., Speller, D.C.E., and Williams, N.B. (1976) Single-dose preoperative antibiotic prophylaxis in gastrointestinal surgery. *Lancet* **ii**, 325–8.
46. Keighley, M.R.B., Crapp, A.R., Burdon, D.W., Cooke, W.T., and Alexander-Williams, J. (1976). Prophylaxis against anaerobic sepsis in bowel surgery. *Br. J. Surg.* **63**, 538–41.
47. Roy, A.D. (1976) The prophylactic use of antimicrobial agents in the surgery of the intestine. *J. antimicrob. Chemother.* **2**, 233–8.
48. Ingham, H.R., Selkon, J.B., So, S.C., and Weiser, R. (1975) Brain abscess. *Br. med. J.* **4**, 39–40.
49. Study Group (1977) Metronidazole in prevention and treatment of bacteroides infections in elective colonic surgery. *Br. med. J.* **1**, 607–10.
50. Ingham, H.R., Rich, G.E., Selkon, J.B., Hale, J.H., Roxby, C.M., Betty, M.J., Johnson, R.W., and Uldall, P.R. (1975) Treatment with metronidazole of three patients with serious infections due to *Bacteroides fragilis*. *J. antimicrob. Chemother.* **1**, 235–42.
51. Eykyn, S.J., and Phillips, I. (1976) Metronidazole and anaerobic sepsis. *Br. med. J.* **4**, 1418–21.

Discussion:

Dr. Simmons: Have you seen bacteroides resistant to metronidazole?

Dr. Willis: Although we have not seen any such bacteroides from clinical material, we have made bacteroides resistant *in vitro*. All our strains have MIC below 5 μg/ml.

Dr. Shanson: We have had a patient at the London Hospital with a bacteroid abdominal sepsis problem from whom we isolated *B. fragilis* with reduced sensitivity—the MIC was 8 μg/ml. This patient had in fact had a course of metronidazole for three months for Crohn's disease.

Dr. Willis: That does not surprise me very much. We have also had a similar case—the patient whose film I showed you earlier with a right-sided subphrenic abscess. That girl had previously had a course of metronidazole for three weeks because of a pelvic abscess with diverticular disease and she has had recurring infection. The organisms we isolated during the second episode were still sensitive.

Dr. Emmerson: We still have problems with inactive discs, in spite of having a bacteroides control. We solve the problem by confirming the tests with another disc when resistance appears to be present.

Dr. Willis: Metronidazole is sensitive to light and Mast Laboratories do not understand this, as the discs are sent out in clear boxes. Most people now use two discs, because they are aware of this. If you store the discs in the dark they should not deteriorate.

Prof. Brumfitt: Could you tell us something about the pharmacokinetics of metronidazole?

Dr. Willis: It is quite a versatile drug. It seems to be absorbed rapidly from wherever you put it. It gets into all tissues including the saliva, mammary secretions and tears, in concentrations about the same as in blood. It crosses the blood–brain barrier without difficulty and it gets into the foetal circulation.

Prof. Brumfitt: Did you mention the bile?

Dr. Willis: It is excreted in the bile, too.

Prof. Asscher: Is there a problem in renal failure?

Dr. Willis: It does not present special problems in renal failure. It is excreted largely in the gut.

Dr. Ridgeway: In view of what we have just heard about partial resistance, are you happy with the use of prophylaxis for 7 days?

Dr. Willis: This depends on your philosophy towards prophylaxis. We are now thinking of lowering the dose and duration.

Dr. Ekland: Is the fluorescence of *B. melanogenicum* more reliable than the pigment formation?

Dr. Willis: Fluorescence will appear in 24 hours but you may have to wait 4 or 5 days for pigmentation. We always look for both. However, you may get a pigmenting organism that doesn't fluoresce.

Dr. Ekland: Is it also dependent on haemoglobin being present in the medium?

Dr. Willis: We always grow it in the presence of haemoglobin, so I can't answer that. But the fluorescing material is not the same as the black pigment.

Prof. O'Grady: It has been suggested that some failure to eradicate vaginal trichomoniasis may be due to degradation of the drug by vaginal flora. If that is a significant factor, one would expect there might be a lot of trouble along those lines with faeces. Could you comment on this?

Dr. Willis: We don't aim to sterilize the gut at all—in fact, we don't think this is possible. We feel that when patients are operated on the important thing is to have circulating drug in their blood so that during operation when you spill organisms into injured tissues, there is the drug there at the time it is needed. One does get degradation in the presence of large numbers of aerobes, but this appears not to matter where one has mixed infections.

Dr. Gaya: Would you care to comment on the adverse effects associated with metronidazole use, and in particular the animal experiments suggesting that it may be a carcinogen and others suggesting that it may be radiosensitizing?

Dr. Willis: I am not competent to discuss the radiosensitization side, but I know that the radiotherapists are very interested. It seems that the drug itself destroys the anaerobic tumour cells rather than being a radiosensitizer. Concerning the carcinogenic effect, there are two papers on this, both from America. One of them says it is carcinogenic and the other says it is not, both on the basis of the same type of experimental data (long-term high-dosage experiments). It is a fact, I gather, that if you reduce the level of food intake of these animals then one gets a 10% increase in the incidence of malignant disease. When you feed animals with metronidazole they automatically reduce their intake by about 5 g a day. So if one puts in a control group on a reduced feeding basis with no drug, you will expect the same incidence of malignant disease.

5

New approaches to the treatment and diagnosis of urinary tract infection

W. BRUMFITT, J.M.T. HAMILTON-MILLER and
S.J.D. BROOKS

One of the major problems concerning the diagnosis and localization of infection in the urinary tract is the lack of standardization of terminology. The Medical Research Council (England) have set up a Sub-Committee on Bacteriuria and, recognizing the confusion which results from terminological misunderstandings, set as one of its objectives a list of precise definitions for many clinical and anatomical terms. However, even if the proposals were to be generally accepted and adopted in Britain, there would still be the problem of gaining their general usage throughout the rest of the world.

For example, 'cystitis' is a widely used term. Its strict medical meaning is 'inflammation of the wall of the bladder'. In fact, patients who complain of 'cystitis' often do not have an inflamed bladder. Furthermore, there is evidence that the symptoms arise from the urethra and bacterial infection may or may not be present. A more logical definition of this symptomatology would be the 'dysuria and frequency syndrome'. Regarding the aetiology, many infecting agents may be found—or none (Figure 1). Perusal of Figure 1 makes it apparent that a patient complaining of dysuria and frequency may be initially referred to one of a number of different hospital departments, such as urology, gynaecology or venereology.

Fig. 1. Microbiological breakdown of 'dysuria/frequency syndrome'

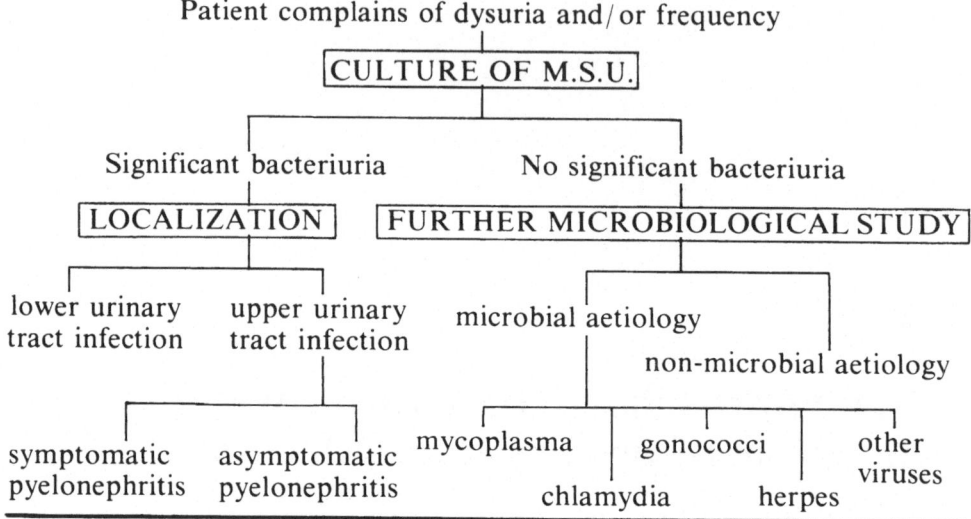

Existing methods of detection of bacteriuria and their shortcomings

Direct (cultural) techniques

Proper microbiological examination of correctly collected freshly voided urine samples enables the distinction to be made between bacteriuria resulting from contamination and infection. Where there is an infection organisms multiply in the bladder urine between successive acts of micturition. Bacterial concentrations are usually in excess of 10^5 organisms per ml of urine. The confidence level rises from 80 to 95% when two (different) consecutive urine specimens are positive.

Quantitative urine culture can be performed by the pour-plate method, but this is time-consuming and expensive. Surface viable counts are easier and widely used for accurate bacterial quantitation for a variety of purposes. Various cheaper and more rapid semi-quantitative - methods have been introduced and these include:

1. Calibrated-loop method. This technique becomes inaccurate if the loop is distorted or is not inserted vertically. Thus, it is too operator-dependent.

2. Filter-paper strip method.

3. Dip-inoculum transport media. This has the added advantage that problems of transport of urine specimens are eliminated. Of the dip-inoculum transport media the most useful is the dip-slide. This may also be inoculated by holding it in the urinary stream—the so-called dip-stream culture. The major disadvantage of this method is that the test is done without dilution of the urine; when confluent growth occurs it can be difficult to assess the significance of the result.

4. Pad culture techniques[1].

Indirect (chemical) techniques

All chemical methods lack sensitivity and specificity and are not, therefore, generally considered suitable for most screening programmes. Kunin and his colleagues [1a], however, claim good results using the nitrite test, although it is inconvenient because at least 3 early morning specimens (EMUs) are needed. Other methods include tests for urinary catalase, the triphenyltetrazolium chloride test and tests for the detection of decreased urinary glucose levels ('Uriglox').

The importance of localization

On a statistical basis it is more difficult to cure upper than lower urinary tract infection. Therefore, failure to distinguish between these sites has resulted in a failure to assess accurately the results of treatment. Other studies have claimed that it is very difficult to classify urinary infections on the basis of symptoms alone [2, 3].

Many techniques have been used for localization of urinary infection [4] but none is entirely satisfactory, nor is there good correlation between different methods. Newer procedures, such as testing for antibody-coated bacteria, have made available an indirect test, causing no discomfort to the patient. This may enable the diagnosis of non-obstructive upper tract disease in women to be made [5]. If this proves to be a reliable method the effect of treatment of upper urinary infection in women will be able to be evaluated with a much greater degree of accuracy, and the importance of renal involvement as a cause of treatment failure more clearly defined. Such information may allow a new approach to be made to these patients, and, by elimination of the infection, prevent progression to more serious forms of renal disease. This would have important economic and social implications.

Infections of the urinary tract are among the commonest infections that afflict humans. In spite of the improvements made in nutrition, hygiene and in the development of more powerful antibiotics, the death rate from infections of the kidneys has not fallen. [6] Nor, after many years of screening programmes, is there any evidence that the incidence of urinary tract infection has fallen [7] or that women attend their general practitioners less often for symptoms of urinary tract infection, or that the incidence of recurrences is less [8-11].

This lack of success is disappointing in view of the progress achieved in other infections, and the improvements in certain areas of urinary tract infections, e.g. the treatment of bacteriuria in pregnancy, to the benefit of both mother and foetus [11a], the awareness of the dangers of catheterization [12, 13], and the institution of 'catheter teams' in paraplegic units [14] and the use of intermittent non-sterile self-catheterization [15].

There is considerable disagreement about how many deaths from infections of the kidney result from repeated or persistent urinary tract infections. Beeson [16] and Heptinstall [17] doubt whether primary infective disease in the adult with healthy kidneys ever results in progression to renal failure. Norden and Kass [18] have stressed that urinary tract infection is so common, and so many adults are affected compared with other kidney diseases, that to evaluate the relative importance of pyelonephritis, not only would a long prospective study of the order of 20 years be necessary, but the numbers would need to be very large. In order to institute screening programmes for adult women a selective approach will be necessary.

Selective screening programmes

The importance of screening pregnant women for asymptomatic bacteriuria is now well established [3, 19] and the need for treatment agreed (although unhappily many workers pay only lip-service to this problem). In some patients the infection is benign, but in others it persists or recurs. [20] In a prospective study, Leigh, Grüneberg and Brumfitt [21] studied 157 women for 2 to 4 years. All these women had asymptomatic bacteriuria in pregnancy and had been treated adequately as judged by proving eradication of the bacteriuria; further, they remained free of infection until six weeks *post partum*. However, 27 relapsed on long-term follow-up. Relapse occurred twice as often among those who had required more than one course of chemotherapy to eradicate the initial bacteriuria. Furthermore, those patients who had been difficult to cure during pregnancy showed a higher incidence of urinary tract abnormalities. No long-term follow-up study has been attempted to see whether it is this group that will be at risk of developing renal failure, and so the actual danger to the individual patient who has had urinary infection during pregnancy remains to be elucidated.

Lindblad and Ekengren [22] have shown that not only is there a high recurrence rate in female children who have urinary tract infection, but that this tendency to relapse remains for many years. In a study extending over 20 years they were able to show that these patients had a high incidence of pyelonephritis in pregnancy.

At present, the consensus of opinion is that the large-scale screening of schoolgirls is not justified, as the incidence of bacteriuria is so low. Also, a high proportion of these bacteriuric children already had renal scarring [1, 23-25]. However, these screening programmes do bring to notice at least some children who are at high risk of recurrent infection and recurrent infection in childhood has been shown to progress to severe renal damage. Animal studies show that the growing kidney is very susceptible to scarring in the presence of bacteria, [26] but the relationship of this observation to the human situation has not been demonstrated in a large-scale study.

At present it would seem that *all* children who have overt or covert infection should be followed over prolonged periods because of their tendency to relapse, especially since the relapse may be asymptomatic. De Wardener [27] estimates that 70 out of 1 000 000 people die from chronic renal failure each year. (Kass [28] doubted this figure.) However, if it is assumed that this is correct and that all died from chronic pyelonephritis, then, on the further assumption that half are female, 35 out of 500 000 die each year. Taking the prevalence of bacteriuria in women to be 5%, of the 500 000 women at risk, 25 000 will be infected. Thus, in the unlikely event (as stated above) that all women who die of renal failure have an infective aetiology, in order to detect one patient progressing to chronic renal failure, 700 patients with bacteriuria would have to be under constant surveillance for at least 20 years. Thus for logistic reasons a non-selective screening approach in women of child-bearing age is clearly impracticable. Screening programmes in adults must be carefully evaluated and directed at high-risk groups, for example those who suffered from urinary infection in pregnancy or have a substantiated history of a previous urinary tract infection.

If large-scale screening programmes for bacteriuria are to be adopted, the method used needs careful evaluation. The dip-slide has proved an effective method for screening on a large scale, but new techniques are becoming available and they will need to be evaluated against the dip-slide in terms of their cost, specificity, sensitivity and predictive value [29]. Our own recent experience with 'Microstix'—a combined culture and nitrite technique—has been encouraging [30].

A comparison between the organisms causing urinary infection in hospital and domiciliary practice is shown in Table 1. It is interesting to note that until recently there did not seem to have been any real change in the relative proportions of different infecting organisms over the years. However, there have now been reports which suggest the emergence of *Micrococcus* spp. as a major urinary tract pathogen, and group B streptococci (*Streptococcus agalactiae*) as a minor one. It may be more than mere coincidence, however, that the increased isolation rate of these two species has come roughly at the same time as the replacement of MacConkey agar by CLED as the primary isolation medium for urine culture. CLED is known to be less inhibitory than MacConkey, so clearly further work must be done to determine whether the apparent change in aetiology is a laboratory artefact.

The various bacterial species isolated from domiciliary patients are more likely to be sensitive to antimicrobial agents. In hospital isolates, resistance to sulphonamides, tetracycline and ampicillin can often be correlated with the usage of the individual agents. In contrast, resistance to trimethoprim does not, in our experience, seem to be increasing, despite the greater use of co-trimoxazole.

Another factor which distinguishes hospital infections from those in domiciliary practice is when cross-infection occurs by highly resistant organisms such as *Serratia marcescens* [31], *Proteus morganii* [32] or *Providencia stuartii* [33]. Under these circumstances, the choice of drugs can be seriously restricted and, in some circumstances, it is impossible to eradicate infection without closing the ward and sterilizing all equipment before recommencing admissions.

Dysuria/frequency syndrome

It is now becoming apparent that a high proportion of these cases are due to microbial aetiology. Dans and Klaus [34] have shown that dysuria and frequency can be caused by gonococci, *Chlamydia trachomatis, Herpesvirus hominis* or candidal vaginitis. This should stimulate the study of the relationship of *Chlamydia* spp., *Ureaplasma urealyticum* (T-strain mycoplasma) and viruses to this syndrome. It is known that dysuria and frequency can precede bacteriuria, but whether any of these other microbial diseases are triggering agents is unknown. Thus, in the dysuria/frequency syndrome without bacterial infection a search should be made for these other organisms, and, if found, appropriate treatment should be given. This is especially true in urethritis in males [35], where *C. trachomatis* has an aetiological role.

Lower urinary tract infection

These infections normally respond rapidly to treatment unless there is some complicating defect, and the bacteriuria can be eradicated by any antibiotic which achieves high urinary levels and is active against the infecting organism (even if the latter appears resistant by the conventional disc test [36]).

Eradication of the lower urinary infection reduces the danger of spread to other parts of the urinary tract, provided that there is no asymptomatic infection elsewhere in the urinary tract, e.g. asymptomatic pyelonephritis or prostatitis. Pyelonephritis is, of course, a special hazard in bacteriuria in pregnancy.

Upper-tract disease

In upper-tract disease the tissue concentration of antibiotics may, in some circumstances, be more important than the urine levels. [37]. There is very little data on the intrarenal distribution of antibiotics. Ampicillin, for example, is said to reach a concentration in the cortex which is twice as high as the concentration in the medulla, and in pyelonephritic kidneys the antibiotic levels in the kidney are half those of serum. [38] However, in medullary infections the concentration in the urine (if diffusion is possible) is more important than blood levels.

Special problems

Infections due to *Proteus* spp. (especially the indole-producing species, which tend to be highly resistant to antibiotics [39]) are difficult to eradicate. The urine becomes very alkaline due to the potent urease produced by these organisms, and is virtually impossible to acidify whilst the organisms are proliferating. Alkaline urine is conducive to the formation of struvite stones [40] inside which bacteria may survive. [41] Analogues of urea, such as acetohydroxamic acid or hydroxyurea, may act as competitive inhibitors of urease. [42, 43] The presence of acetohydroxamate in urine allows stone dissolution to occur experimentally; [40] however, clinical trials in man will probably be considerably delayed because of the alleged carcinogenicity of hydroxamate. This type of new approach may greatly simplify problems of long-term prophylaxis (see below). It should be pointed out that several other urinary tract pathogens, such as klebsiellae, micrococci and T-strain mycoplasmas, also produce urease and some of these have been shown to produce stones clinically [41] or in the animal model. [44] The importance of the prostate as a source of infection in the male should be remembered. Prostatitis is an obvious reservoir for infection leading to recurrent pyelonephritis, and bears some similarity to recurrent attacks of dysuria/frequency syndrome. [45] The problem is much increased when calculi develop in the prostate. The main difficulty in reviewing the literature is that various definitions of the condition have been used. Great attention must be paid to obtaining proper specimens and processing them correctly. Thus, Stamey [46] has stressed the importance of using the first 10 ml of urine passed as a maximal volume suitable for study. He also stresses the need to use an inoculum of more than 0.1 ml on the plate, in order not to fail to detect small numbers of significant organisms. Infection is difficult to eradicate in chronic prostatic infection because many antimicrobial agents are lipophobic, bind to proteins and are highly ionized in the plasma. [46] However, trimethoprim reaches high levels in the prostate, and this offers hope either of complete cure or, if this is not possible, its use as a long-term prophylactic agent. Erythromycin is another antibiotic which penetrates the prostate, but is of limited use due to its relatively narrow spectrum of activity, although it may have a place in chronic prostatitis when the prostate is colonized by mixed organisms, including staphylococci. Thus, it is important to appreciate that Gram-positive organisms may be important pathogens in chronic prostatitis. In the past some workers (including ourselves) have been guilty of dismissing small numbers of such organisms as saprophytes, whereas we now realize their pathogenic role in prostatitis. Chloramphenicol and lincomycin are other antibacterial agents which should pass into the prostate, but each has obvious limitations.

Prostatic infections cause the excretion of antibody-coated bacteria, and it has been suggested that this may prove to be a useful diagnostic tool for demonstrating tissue infection as well as being an index of the effectiveness of treatment. [47]

Dose of antimicrobial agent

All dosages of antibacterial agents used in urinary tract infection are virtually chosen on a completely arbitrary basis. There seems to have been little or no effort made to establish what the *minimum* curative dose of an antibiotic is, or what the optimal method or period for its administration should be. For instance, sulphadimidine is still prescribed on a 6-hourly schedule, when its half-life is in the order of 17 hours. Sulphadimidine is classified by the Food and Drugs Administration as a standard for a 'short-acting sulphonamide' (I. Lenox-Smith, personal communication). This situation presumably exists because sulphonamides have been in use since the late 1930s when the concept of pharmacokinetics as a guide to dosage was very hazy. The dose schedule initially adopted, which proved to be clinically effective, has not been changed in the light of more recently acquired knowledge. Another example of a compound that may be being given in an inappropriate dosage schedule is nitrofurantoin, for which pharmacokinetic studies are still in an unsatisfactory state. [48]

There is a tacit assumption that in the treatment of urinary tract infection optimal results will be obtained by keeping as high a level as possible of the antibacterial agent in the urine for a period of one week. On the other hand, permanent removal of bacteria might sometimes be more rapid if lower levels were maintained (as our own recent experiments [49] indicate in a special case). These important problems need careful study; possible reductions in antibiotic dosage in urinary tract infection would be an advantage to the patient in terms of side-effects, toxicity, convenience and cost, and to the environment in terms of reduced exposure.

The development of local antiseptics and their use in the introital area has had some success, although the experimental design was poor [50, 51], and it is surprising that such an obvious approach has not had more attention. These studies are interesting but somewhat superficial, making it difficult to draw firm conclusions about the use of local agents in this context, and wider trials are clearly required. The whole topic of introital colonization suffers from the defect that there is little standardization in methods of sampling and quantitation. We hope that the new approach proposed and tried by us [52] will prove to be successful.

Very little is known about the flora of the periurethral area and its variation in normal women, so that abnormal findings are difficult to define.

Where antiseptics and prophylactic therapy prove inadequate, then there may be a place for levamisole, which stimulates the local production of IgA. This drug was introduced first as an antihelminthic, but it has the effect of stimulating local immunity, and has been used in recurrent herpes [53] and recurrent respiratory tract infections in children. [54]

Duration of treatment

For treatment of an acute infection it is our practice to prescribe a seven-day course of treatment. Great emphasis is placed upon pre-treatment diagnosis and proof of cure by follow-up one week and five weeks after the end of treatment.

It must be admitted that choice and duration of treatment are arbitrary. As will be seen below, many factors influence treatment. For example, a recent study of the dysuria/frequency syndrome in domiciliary practice, using amoxycillin, showed no difference between a 3- and 10-day course. [55]

On the other hand, treatment of asymptomatic bacteriuria in pregnancy with a five-day course of ampicillin gave inferior results to a ten-day course. [56] Similarly, Kincaid-Smith and Fairley [57] could find no improvement by prolonging a 2-week course of ampicillin to 6 weeks.

The question arises here as to the degree of patient compliance; little has been published about this in relation to the treatment of urinary tract infections, although it is known that, in general, compliance for antibiotics is bad. [58] Workers in Germany [59] found, in a recent large study, no antibacterial activity in the urine of 27% of patients who had been prescribed antibiotic treatment.

The once popular practice of giving antibiotics in therapeutic dosage for 6 months, or even changing the antibiotic every month, has now been discarded by serious workers. Such methods have no advantage, may disguise a latent infection and increase the risk of toxicity and side-effects, whilst at the same time selecting for resistance in the bowel flora. In reduced dosage, however, prophylactic antimicrobial therapy has been very successful (see below).

Attempts to treat patients with a single large dose of a bactericidal antibiotic have not been successful [60, 61] and by contrast, the use of an ultra long-acting compound (sulfadoxine) gave results similar to those with a 7-day course of ampicillin, when a comparison was made in domiciliary practice [62]—a surprising finding. Unfortunately, this compound has now been withdrawn because of the suspicions that it may cause erythema multiforme, especially where there was prolonged exposure to hot sun.

Renal calculus

This problem is a very serious one. [46] The role of surgical treatment has been doubted in recent years because of the high rate of recurrence. Thus, the major problem seems to be that minute stones remain after surgery, and persistent infections by urea-splitting organisms recur. This has resulted in attempts to treat the condition medically, using Renacidin (a mixture of organic acids) infused into the renal pelvis post-operatively. However, great care must be taken since, if the pressure rises above that of the venous pressure, reverse flow can occur into the vascular system with disastrous results (i.e. death). The use of this procedure can therefore only be considered in highly specialized urological departments.

Clearly, the problem of stone remains a major one causing much severe morbidity, and, in some cases, mortality. The most promising development in this field is the work on inhibitors of urease and oxalate-forming precursors.

Chronic bacteriuria

Chronic bacteriuria can arise in different ways. For example, abnormalities of bladder emptying as well as bladder diverticula result in residual urine and allow small numbers of bacteria to gain access to the bladder to become established and remain for a long period of time. Some women suffer repeated episodes of dysuria/frequency syndrome over a number of years and become debilitated and demoralized by their illness, even though no serious organic lesion can be recognized. Most of these problems are seen in domiciliary practice, and in those with infection the problem is usually one of recurrent reinfection from outside the urinary tract rather than persistent infection within the urinary tract. [9] Some of the patients are unfortunate enough to end in the hands of the psychiatrist—truly a tragic fate.

Nevertheless, both in children and adults a proportion of the patients is liable not only to infection of the bladder urine but also of the renal parenchyma. There is some evidence to suggest that this situation is especially dangerous in female children with persistent infection accompanied by uretero-vesical reflux.

The treatment of chronic bacteriuria is extremely controversial. There is no general agreement about how often chronic bacteriuria confined to the lower urinary tract ascends to involve the kidney. In children and in pregnant women there is strong evidence that there is a substantial risk of kidney involvement with serious complications, so that treatment should always be given. In the elderly with chronic bacteriuria views on the need for long-term therapy differ but treatment is always needed if the patient is symptomatic or showing deterioration in renal function.

The antimicrobial agent used must have low toxicity and have minimal side-effects. It must also not affect the bowel flora or predispose to the selection of bacteria harbouring R-factors, which are liable to cause 'breakthrough infections'. Successful results have been obtained with methenamine mandelate together with urinary acidification. [63, 64] Alternative treatments have been used: co-trimoxazole [65, 66] or nitrofurantoin. [67] Cephalexin given in small doses (presumably to prevent selection of R-factors in the colonic enterobacteria) has been reported to be an effective prophylactic agent. [68]

When methenamine mandelate or nitrofurantoin is used for prophylactic regimens, the problem caused by organisms that alkalinize the urine (see above) is a serious one (Brumfitt, Cooper and Brooks, unpublished data). However, in view of experimental evidence using a mixture of methenamine and acetohydroxamic acid [69], this problem may be overcome in the near future. At the present time we are investigating the use of a low dose of trimethoprim, which has been used successfully by others (e.g. [70]) This used alone does not appear to give rise to resistant variants in the bowel, and the small tablet is highly acceptable to the patient. A further advantage of either co-trimoxazole or trimethoprim is that these compounds can be used in patients with chronic renal failure, provided that the dose is adjusted according to the degree of impaired kidney function. [71, 72] We have found trimethoprim to be excreted in the vaginal secretions, and this compound reduces the number of *Esch. coli* in the bowel flora. These properties may be valuable in eliminating or preventing colonization of the introitus which we have found to be an important precipitating cause of recurrent urinary tract infection.

Rationale of laboratory tests

We have already alluded to the fact that cure rates for urinary tract infection, and the death rate from pyelonephritis, have remained largely unchanged for the past 20–25 years. The latter is not so surprising, as there must be a very long lag period before an improvement could be seen. However, the lack of progress in curing urinary tract infection is much more serious, especially in view of general advances in the field, such as the introduction of antibacterial compounds such as ampicillin and co-trimoxazole. Diagnostic procedures (dip-slide screening in pregnancy, localization studies) and epidemiological investigations have been referred to above. Distinction between reinfection and relapse is also crucial. [73] Also, in other bacterial infections (e.g. pneumonia and some common varieties of meningitis) cure rates have increased and death rates decreased. It is particularly distressing since, *prima facie*, urinary tract infection should be much easier than other microbial infections to treat, because of the highly favourable pharmacokinetic situation, with the antibiotic being concentrated at the site of infection. The unsatisfactory situation must be explicable in terms of host, parasite, clinical management and laboratory factors. The first three factors have been described above, and it does not seem on the balance that lack of progress can be blamed upon any one of them.

Several questions do arise, however, when laboratory techniques are looked at closely. For instance, what is the validity of carrying out a conventional disc test for sensitivity on a rich, complex medium? Urine is a relatively poor medium which is liquid, contains much urea (a potent antibacterial agent)[74]—and is of highly variable pH, osmolality and ionic strength; yet the results of disc tests are often extrapolated directly, without questioning, to the clinical situation. Again, MIC testing, carried out by the tube method, requires the growth of at least 10^7 bacteria/ml before being scored as positive (viz. turbid to the naked eye); 10^5 organisms/ml—representing a 'significant bacteriuria' [19]— would be scored as 'no growth' using the turbidity method. The question of inoculum size is crucial in the testing of such compounds as sulphonamides and trimethoprim; the best inoculum to use for laboratory purposes is 10^4 bacteria per plate. If the inoculum exceeds this number 'sensitive' strains appear to be 'resistant'. How does this latter finding apply to conditions in the bladder during a urinary tract infection when concentrations are known to exceed 10^7/ml in urine? The precise role played in urinary tract infection, especially the relapsing kind, of organisms which can take on a defective, persisting form (e.g. L-forms, cystine-requiring or thymine-dependent strains) will not be uncovered until all specimens can be processed in such a way that this type of organism can be detected using a method which has real potential clinical relevance. This will be an expensive and time-consuming extra work-load for the routine laboratory, but in the end will lead to better methods, to the benefit of everyone.

Table 1. 1000 consecutive isolates from hospital and domiciliary practice (from Brumfitt (1974), ref. 4)

Organism	Domiciliary %	Hospital %
Escherichia coli	90	59
Proteus spp.	5 (mirabilis)	16
Klebsiella-Enterobacter	2	9
staphylococci	3 (albus)	5
Pseudomonas aeruginosa	—	3
streptococci	—	7
Miscellaneous	—	1
Total strains studied	1000	1000

References

1. Kunin. C.M.. Deutscher. R.. and Paquin. A. (1964) Urinary tract infection in school children: an epidemiologic and clinical laboratory study. *Medicine, Baltimore* **43**. 91–130.

1a. Brumfitt. W.. Percival. A. and Williams. J.D. (1973) Estimation of bacteria and white cells in the urine. *ACP Broadsheet* no. 80.

2. Gallagher, D.J.A., Montgomerie, J.Z., and North, J.D.K. (1965) Acute infections of the urinary tract and the urethral syndrome in general practice. *Br. med. J.* **1**, 622–6.

3. Williams, J.D., Leigh, D.A., Rosser, A. ap I., and Brumfitt, W. (1965) The organization and results of a screening programme for the detection of bacteriuria of pregnancy. *J. Obstet. Gynaecol. Brit. Commonw*. **72**, 327–35.

4. Brumfitt. W. (1972) Bacteriological aspects of renal disease. In *Renal disease*, 367–97, ed. Black, D.A.K., 3rd edn. Blackwell. Oxford.

5. Thomas, V.L., Shelokov, A., and Forland. M. (1974) Antibody-coated bacteria in the urine and the site of urinary tract infection. *New Engl. J. Med.* **290**, 588–90.

6. Registrar-General's Statistical Review of England and Wales for 1973–4. Her Majesty's Stationery Office 1975.

7. Hospital In-Patient Enquiry for 1971. Department of Health and Social Security and Office of Population Census and Surveys. Stationery Office, 1973.

8. Fry, J.. Dillane, J.B., Joiner, C.L., and Williams, J.D. (1962) Acute urinary infections: their course and outcome in general practice with special reference to chronic pyelonephritis. *Lancet* **i**, 1318–21.

9. Mond, N.C., Percival, A., Williams, J.D., and Brumfitt, W. (1965) Presentation, diagnosis and treatment of urinary tract infections in general practice. *Lancet* **i**, 514–16.

10. Asscher, A.W., Sussman, M., Waters, W.E., Evans, J.A.S., Campbell, H., Evans, K.T., and Williams, J.E. (1969) Asymptomatic significant bacteriuria in the non-pregnant woman. *Br. med. J.* **1**, 804–6.

11. Lawson, D.H., Clarke, A.. McFarlane. D.B., McAllister, T.A. and Linton, A.L. (1973) Urinary tract symptomatology in general practice. *J. Roy. Coll. General Practitioners* **23**, 548-55.

11a. Brumfitt. W. (1975) The effects of bacteriuria in pregnancy on maternal and fetal health. *Kidney International* **8**. 113–9.

12. Brumfitt, W., Davies, B.I., and Rosser, E. ap I. (1961) Urethral catheter as a cause of urinary tract infection in pregnancy and puerperium. *Lancet* ii, 1059–62.
13. Beeson, P.B. (1958) The case against the catheter. *Am. J. Med.* **24**, 1–3.
14. Pearman, J.W., and England, E.J. (1973) *Urological management of the patient following spinal cord injury.* Thomas, Springfield, Ill.
15. Editorial (1976) Intermittent non-sterile self-catheterization. *Br. med. J.* **2**, 5–6.
16. Beeson, P.B. (1967) Urinary tract infection and pyelonephritis. In *Renal disease*, 382–403, ed. Black, D.A.K., 2nd edn. Blackwell, Oxford.
17. Heptinstall, R.H. (1967) The limitations of the pathological diagnosis of chronic pyelonephritis. In *Renal disease*, 350–81, ed. Black, D.A.K., 2nd edn. Blackwell, Oxford.
18. Norden, C.W., and Kass, E.H. (1968) Bacteriuria of pregnancy—a critical appraisal. *Ann. Rev. Med.* **19**, 431–70.
19. Kass, E.H. (1956) Asymptomatic infections of the urinary tract. *Trans. Ass. Am. Physicians* **69**, 56–64.
20. Brumfitt, W., Grüneberg, R.N., and Leigh, D.A. (1967) Bacteriuria in pregnancy: with reference to prematurity and long-term effects on the matter. In *Symposium on pyelonephritis*, 20–27. E. and S. Livingstone, Edinburgh.
21. Leigh, D.A., Grüneberg, R.N., and Brumfitt, W. (1968) Long-term follow-up of bacteriuria in pregnancy. *Lancet* i, 603–5.
22. Lindblad, B.S., and Ekengren, K. (1969) The long-term prognosis of non-obstructive urinary tract infection in infancy and childhood after the advent of sulphonamides. *Acta paediat. Scand.* **58**, 25–32.
23. Savage, D.C.L., Howie, G., Adler, K., and Wilson, M.I. (1975) Controlled trial of therapy in covert bacteriuria of childhood. *Lancet* i, 358–61.
24. Savage, D.C.L., Wilson, M.I., McHardy, M., Dewar, D.A.E., and Fee, W.M. (1973) Covert bacteriuria in childhood: a clinical and epidemiological study. *Arch. Dis. Childh.* **48**, 8–20.
25. Asscher, A.W. (1976) Round Table Discussion. In *Urinary Tract Infection* 25–26, eds. Brumfitt, W., and Asscher, A.W. Oxford University Press, London.
26. Asscher, A.W., Chick, S., Roberts, E.M., Evans, K.T., and Williams, J.E. (1970) Effect of ascending *Escherichia coli* infection on compensatory hypertrophy of the rat kidney. In *Renal infection and renal scarring*, 303–13, eds. Kincaid-Smith, P., and Fairley, K.F. Mercedes, Australia.
27. de Wardener, H.E. (1967) *The Kidney: an outline of normal and abnormal structure and function,* 3rd edn. J. and A. Churchill, London.
28. Kass, E.H., (1969) Discussion in 'Symposium on Pyelonephritis'. *J. infect. Dis.* **120**, 1–140.
29. Krieg, A.G., Gambino, R., and Galen, R.S. (1975) Why are clinical laboratory tests performed? When are they valid? *J. Am. med. Ass.* **223**, 75–8.
30. Hamilton-Miller, J.M.T., Brooks, S.J.D., Brumfitt, W., and Bakhtiar, M. (1977) Screening for bacteriuria: Microstix and dip-slides. *Postgrad. med. J.* **53**, 248–50.
31. Madduri, S.D., Mauriello, D.A., Smith, L.G., and Seebode, J.J. (1976) *Serratia marcescens* and the urologist. *J. Urol.* **116**, 613–15.
32. Lindsey, J.O., Martin, W.T., Sonnenwirth, A.C., and Bennett, J.V., (1976) An outbreak of nosocomial *Proteus rettgeri* urinary tract infection. *Am. J. Epidemiol.* **103**, 261–9.
33. Overturf, G.D. Wilkins, J., and Ressler, R. (1974) Emergence of resistance of *Providencia stuartii* to multiple antibiotics: speciation and biochemical characterization of *Providencia*. *J. infect. Dis.* **129**, 353–7.
34. Dans, P.E., and Klaus, B. (1976) Dysuria in women. *Johns Hopkins med. J.* **138**, 13–18.
35. Holmes, K.K., Handsfield, H.H., Wang, S.P., Wentworth, B.B., Turck, M., Anderson, J.B., and Alexander, E.R. (1975) Etiology of nongonococcal urethritis. *New Engl. J. Med.* **292**, 1199–205.

36. Musher, D.M. Minuth, J.N., Thorsteinsson, S.B., and Holmes, T. (1975) Effectiveness of achievable urinary concentrations of tetracyclines against 'tetracycline-resistant' pathogenic bacteria. *J. infect. Dis.* **131**, S40–S44.
37. Whelton, A., and Walker, W.G. (1974) Intrarenal antibiotic distribution in health and disease. *Kidney International* **6**, 131–7.
38. Whelton, A., Sapir, D.G., Carter, G.G., Garth, M.A., and Walker, W.G. (1972) Intrarenal distribution of ampicillin in the normal and diseased human kidney. *J. infect. Dis.* **125**, 466–70.
39. Fiedelman, W. (1975) Carbenicillin therapy of urinary tract infections due to difficult uropathogens. *Curr. Therap. Res.* **18**, 257–9.
40. Griffith, D.P., Musher, D.M., and Itin, C. (1976) Urease. The primary cause of infection-induced urinary stones. *Invest. Urol.* **13**, 346–50.
41. Nemoy, N.J., and Stamey, T.A. (1971) Surgical, bacteriological and biochemical management of 'infection stones'. *J. Am. med. Ass.* **215**, 1470–6.
42. Griffith, D., Musher, D.M., and Campbell, J.W. (1973) Inhibition of bacterial urease. *Invest. Urol.* **11**, 228–33.
43. Aronson, M., Medalia, O., and Griffel, B. (1974) Prevention of ascending pyelonephritis in mice by urease inhibitors. *Nephron* **12**, 94–104.
44. Friedlander, A.M., and Braude, A.I. (1974) Production of bladder-stones by human T mycoplasmas. *Nature, Lond.* **247**, 67–9.
45. Moore, T. (1968) The urethra in relation to recurrent infection. In *Urinary tract infection*, 187–93, eds. O'Grady, F., and Brumfitt, W. Oxford University Press.
46. Stamey, T.A., (1972) *Urinary infections.* Williams and Wilkins Co., Baltimore.
47. Jones, S.R. (1974) Prostatitis as a cause of antibody-coated bacteria in urine. *New Engl. J. Med.* **291**, 365.
48. Hamilton-Miller, J.M.T., Kerry, D.W., Reynolds, A., and Brumfitt, W. (1977) Two new bioassay techniques for nitrofurans: *Bacteroides fragilis* and *rec. Escherichia coli* as indicator strains. *Chemotherapy* **23**, 236–42.
49. Kerry, D.W., Hamilton-Miller, J.M.T., and Brumfitt, W. (1976) Paradoxical effect of mecillinam on *Providencia stuartii. J. antimicrob. Chemother.* **2**, 386–8.
50. Landes, R.R., Melnick, I., and Hoffman, A.A. (1970) Recurrent urinary tract infections in women. *J. Urol.* **104**, 749–50.
51. Jameson, R.M. (1976) The prevention of recurrent urinary tract infection in woman. *Practitioner* **216**, 178–81.
52. Brumfitt, W., Hamilton-Miller, J.M.T., Bakhtiar, M,. and Cooper, J. (1976) New technique for investigating bacteriai flora of female periurethal area. *Br. med. J.* **2**, 1471-2
53. Kint, A., and Verlinden L. (1974) Levamisole for recurrent *herpes labialis. New Engl. J. Med.* **291**, 308.
54. Van Eygen, M., Znamensky, P.Y., Meck, E., and Raymaekers, I. (1976) Levamisole in prevention of recurrent upper respiratory tract infections in children. *Lancet* i, 382–5.
55. Charlton, C.A.C., Crowther, A., Davies, J.G., Dynes, J., Haward, M.W.A., Mann, P.G., and Rye, S. (1976) Three-day and ten-day chemotherapy for urinary tract infections in general practice. *Br. med. J.* **1**, 124–6.
56. Brumfitt, W., Percival, A., and Carter, M.J. (1962) Treatment of urinary tract infections with ampicillin: a clinical trial. *Lancet* i, 130–3.
57. Kincaid-Smith, P., and Fairley, K.F. (1969) Controlled trial comparing effect of two and six weeks' treatment in recurrent urinary tract infection. *Br. med. J.* **2**, 145–6.
58. Sharpe, T., and Mikeal, R. (1974) Patient compliance with antibiotic regimens. *Am. J. Hosp. Pharmacy* **31**, 479–84.
59. Ansorg, R., Zappel, H., and Thomssen, R. (1975) Bedeutung des Nachweises antibakterieller Stoffe im Urin fur die bakteriologische Diagnostik und die Kontrolle der Chemotherapie von Harnwegsinfektionen. *Zbl. Bakt. Hyg.* **1**, Abt.

Orig. A **230**, 492–507.

60. Brumfitt, W., Faiers, M.C., and Franklin, I.N.S. (1970) The treatment of urinary infection by means of a single dose of cephaloridine. *Postgrad. med. J.* **46**, (Suppl.), 65–8.

61. Grüneberg, R.N., Smellie, J.M., Leakey, A., and Atkin, W.S. (1976) Long-term low-dose co-trimoxazole in prophylaxis of childhood urinary tract infection: Bacteriological aspects. *Br. med. J.* **2**, 206–8.

62. Grüneberg, R.N. and Brumfitt, W. (1967) Single dose treatment of urinary tract infection: a controlled trial. *Br. med. J.* **3**, 649–51.

63. Brumfitt, W., Pursell, R., Franklin, I., and Davies, B.I.D. (1974) Prevention of recurrent urinary infection in females by prophylactic chemotherapy (methenamine mandelate) with or without diuresis. In *Progress in chemotherapy*, Vol. 2, 699–704, ed. Daikos, G. Hellenic Society of Chemotherapy.

64. Freeman, R.B., Smith, W.M., Richardson, J.A., Hennelly, P.J., Thurm, R.H., Urner, C., Vaillancourt, J.A., Griep, R.J., and Bromer, L. (1975) Long-term therapy for chronic bacteriuria in men. *Ann. intern. Med.* **83**, 133–47.

65. Williams, J.D., and Smith, E.K. (1970) Single-dose therapy with streptomycin and sulfametopyrazine for bacteriuria in pregnancy. *Br. med. J.* **4**, 651–3.

66. Stamey, T.A., Condy, M., and Mihara, G. (1977) Prophylactic efficacy of nitrofurantoin macrocrystals and trimethoprim-sulfamethoxazole in urinary infections. *New Engl. J. Med.* **4**, 780–3.

67. Lippman, R.W., Wrobel, C.J., Rees, R., and Hoyt, R. (1958) A theory concerning recurrence of urinary infection: prolonged administration of nitrofurantoin for prevention. *J. Urol.* **80**, 77–81.

68. Gower, P.E. (1975) The use of small doses of cephalexin (125 mg) in the management of recurrent urinary tract infection in women. *J. antimicrob. Chemother.* **1**, (Suppl.), 93–8.

69. Musher, D.M. Griffith, D.P., Tyler, M., and Woelfel, A. (1974) Potentiation of the antibacterial effect of methenamine by acetohydroxamic acid. *Antimicrob. Agents Chemother.* **5**, 101–5.

70. Kasanen, A., Kaarsalo, E., Hiltunen, R., and Soini, V. (1974) Comparison of long-term, low-dosage nitrofurantoin, methenamine hippurate, trimethoprim and trimethoprim-sulphamethoxazole on the control of recurrent urinary tract infection. *Annls clin. Res.* **6**, 285–9.

71. Whelton, A. (1974) Antibacterial chemtherapy in renal insufficiency: a review. *Antibiotica et Chemotherapia* **18**, 1–48.

72. Tasker, P.R.W., MacGregor, G.A., de Wardener, H.E., Thomas, R.D., and Jones, N.F. (1975) Use of co-trimoxazole in chronic renal failure. *Lancet* **i**, 1216–18.

73. Grüneberg, R.N. Leigh, D.A. and Brumfitt, W. (1968) *Escherichia coli* serotypes in urinary tract infection: studies in domiciliary ante-natal and hospital practice. In *Urinary Tract Infection* 68–79, eds. O'Grady, F. and Brumfitt, W. Oxford University Press, London.

74. Schlegel, J.U., Cuellar, J., and O'Dell, R.M. (1961) Bactericidal effect of urea. *J. Urol.* **86**, 819–22.

Discussion

Prof. Asscher: You say in Cardiff we have been accused of saying that 'it is not worth treating bacteriuria in pregnancy' which is a misreading of all that we have ever written! I agree with you that treatment of bacteriuria in pregnancy is mandatory. In contrast, as far as the natural history in non-pregnant women is concerned, what you did not mention is that we have followed up 700–800 women for a period of up to 12 years. Despite their radiological abnormalities, unless there was gross obstruction, they had not actually got worse without any treatment. Thus, the reason for this theoretical argument was to show that it is obviously not possible to prove the absence of deterioration but that it is a great rarity to see progressive disease of the kidneys in adult women in the absence of obstruction. If you are talking in public health terms (value for money) screening is unlikely to succeed.

Prof. Brumfitt: All I was trying to say was that you could possibly prevent recurrent infections by long-term therapy. I agree that hard evidence of progressive renal disease in non-pregnant women with urinary infection is lacking.

Dr. Percival: You said that it was possible to measure the level of antibiotics and IgA in vaginal secretions. How is this done?

Prof. Brumfitt: Simply by using pre-weighed polystyrene sponges and eluting the material in the secretions and doing fluorescent studies by appropriate methods.

Dr. Lowry: Is it necessary to acidify the urine when using Mandelamine?

Prof. Brumfitt: With Mandelamine it now seems that the pH need not be reduced as much as we had previously thought necessary. A level of the order of 6.5 seems to be all right. We use 4 g a day of Mandelamine. More recently, we have been using Hiprex 1 g twice daily with no acidification with good results. We are trying to discover why such a low dose without acidification is effective.

6

Role of complement in infectious disease

M.B. PEPYS

The complement system

Complement is a complex system of plasma proteins which have diverse interactions with other plasma proteins, including antibodies (immunoglobulins) and the coagulation system, as well as with all types of leucocytes. Many of the complement components are synthesized by cells of the monocyte/macrophage line (Table 1) [1], and the structural genes for some of them are located near the major histocompatibility locus [2,3]. Most of the complement proteins exist in the native state in the plasma as proenzymes which upon activation acquire both enzymatic activity and the capacity to bind to, or become fixed upon, suitable acceptor sites such as cell surfaces or macromolecular protein aggregates [4]. Once fixed the components express their enzymatic activity, frequently upon the next component in the sequence. The process of activation usually involves splitting of the molecule and both the split fragment in solution and the fixed activated fragment may have distinct biological activities [4]. There are

Table 1.   Sites of formation of complement components

Classical pathway	*Site*
C1	Macrophages/monocytes ? Intestinal epithelium
C4	Macrophages/monocytes
C2	Macrophages/monocytes
C3	Macrophages/monocytes Hepatocytes
C5	Macrophages/monocytes Hepatocytes
C6	Liver
C7	?
C8	?Spleen
C9	Liver
Alternative pathway	
B	Macrophages ?lymphocytes
D, P, C3NeF, etc.	?
Inhibitors	
C1 inhibitor	Liver
C3b (C4) INA	?

complex and subtle control mechanisms of enzymatic and stoichiometric inhibitors and inactivators which regulate complement activation and the expression of biological activity by its products (Figure 1) [4, 5].

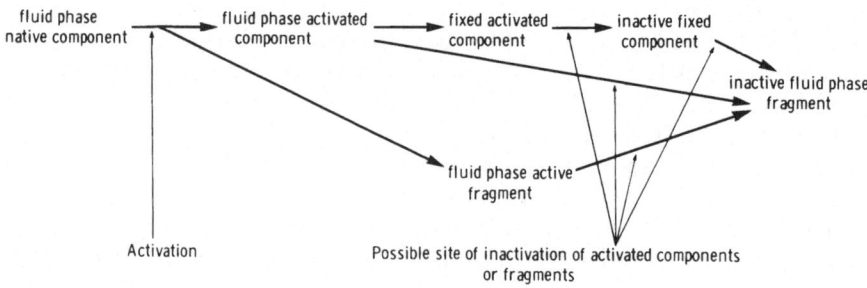

Figure 1. Functional characteristics of the complement system

There are at least three major pathways, involving different early components, by which complement can be activated and thereby express its functions, and these pathways are initiated by different activators via distinct mechanisms (Figure 2) [4]. The biological consequences of complement activation fall into three main groups:

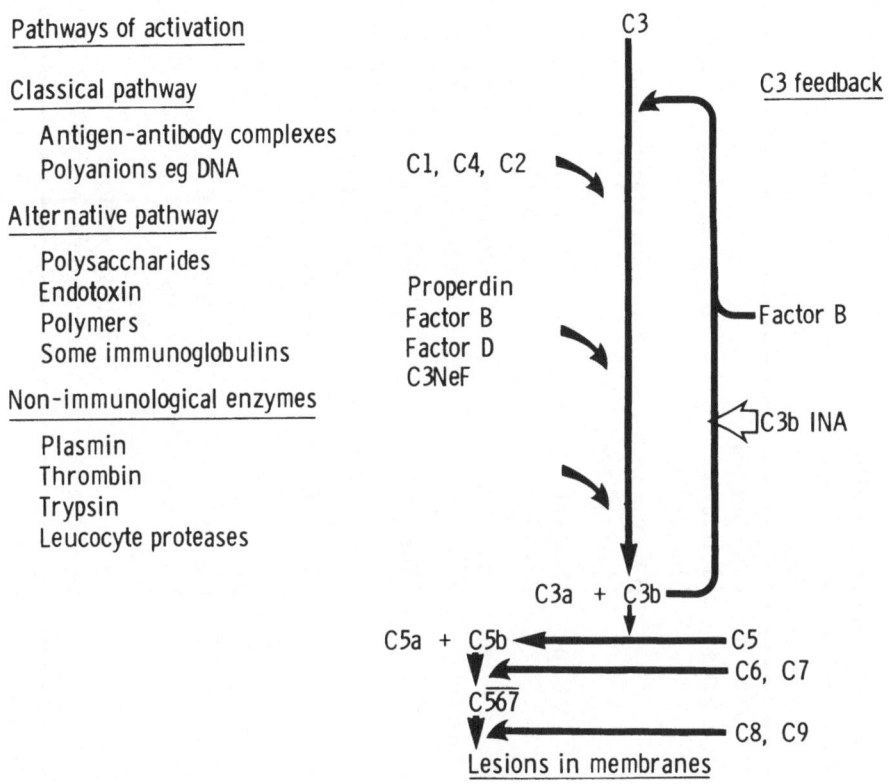

Figure 2. Complement

i. fixed complement, chiefly C3, is responsible for cellular adherence reactions;

ii. fluid-phase and fixed complement fragments can convey triggering signals to certain cells, thereby initiating particular cellular activities;

iii. fixation of the terminal 'attack' sequence of complement components C5–C9 upon cell membranes producing membrane lesions (Table 2) [4, 6]. All the different pathways of activation and varieties of

Table 2. Biological consequences of complement activation

Function	Mechanism	Cells	Effect
Adherence	Binding of fixed C3 to cell surface C3 receptors	Polymorphs Monocytes Macrophages	Adherence for phagocytosis
		B lymphocytes Macrophages	?Antigen presentation
Trigger signal	Recognition of C3a, C5a at cell surface	Mast cells Basophils	Degranulation releasing bioactive amines
	Recognition of C3a, C5a, C$\overline{5}$67 at cell surface	Phagocytic cells	Directed migration of neutrophils, monocytes, eosinophils
	Binding of fixed or fluid phase C3b	Phagocytes	?Activation of lysosomes ?Enhanced intracellular killing ?Trigger to phagocytosis
		?B lymphocytes	Release of monocyte chemotactic factor
Membrane lesions	Fixation of C5–C9 on cell membranes	Blood cells Platelets Nucleated cells Microorganisms	Lysis Release of PF3 Lysis Lysis Killing without lysis
		Solid organs	Lysosomal activation

biological effects are relevant to the role of complement in infectious disease.

Many aspects of the complement system, its genetics, pathways and molecular basis of activation and effects, and its clinical relevance, have been the subject of extensive research in the past few years. Examples of important new concepts have been:

i. antibody-independent complement activation by biopolymers and other biological macromolecules [7, 8];

ii. the C3-feedback loop [9];

iii. interaction with other plasma enzyme systems [10] and with phagocytic cells [11];

iv. participation in lymphoid tissue function [12];

v. the induction of antibody production [13, 14].

This chapter will review only a few selected topics with the aim of illustrating participation of complement both in protective immunity to microorganisms and in mediating the hypersensitivity reactions which underlie many important manifestations of infectious disease.

Complement in immunity

A major function of the complement system is its participation in the activities of phagocytic cells. The split fragments C3a [15] and C5a [16, 17], and the fluid-phase complex C567 [18] are among the most potent and important chemotactic stimuli generated in foci of inflammation. Their presence leads to the accumulation in these foci of neutrophils and other phagocytes. Interaction of fixed C3b on complement-coated particles with receptors for it (which are present on neutrophils and monocyte/macrophages) greatly enhances the adherence to cell surfaces which is a prerequisite for ingestion [11, 19-24] (Figure 3). Furthermore there is now evidence that this interaction, and even the binding of unfixed, fluid-phase C3b, may 'activate' macrophages [25, 26] and thereby increase their capacity for killing ingested microorganisms. Fixation of the terminal complement components on cell membranes, including those of some microorganisms, produces membrane damage which can lyse cells or even kill without lysis [4] (Figure 4). This is probably not a major mechanism of protective immunity since the rare individuals with genetic deficiency of one or other of the late components (C5–C9) do not seem to be unduly susceptible to infection except possibly by *Neisseria* species [27]. In marked contrast patients with genetic deficiencies of the complement system which interfere with their capacity to activate and fix C3 suffer from severe immunity deficiency characterized by repeated bacterial infections, and resemble individuals with antibody-deficiency syndrome [27].

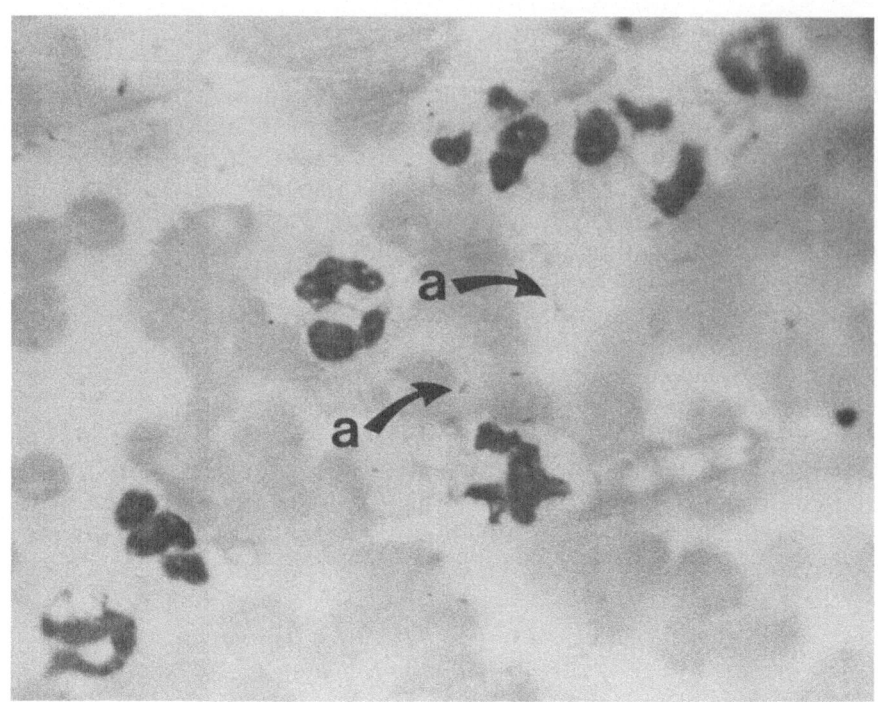

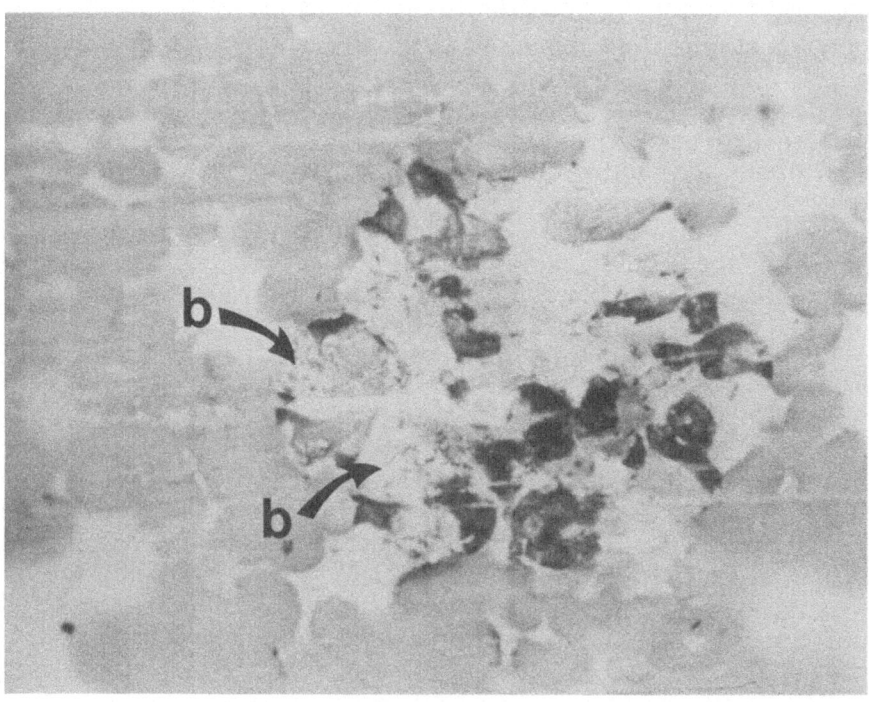

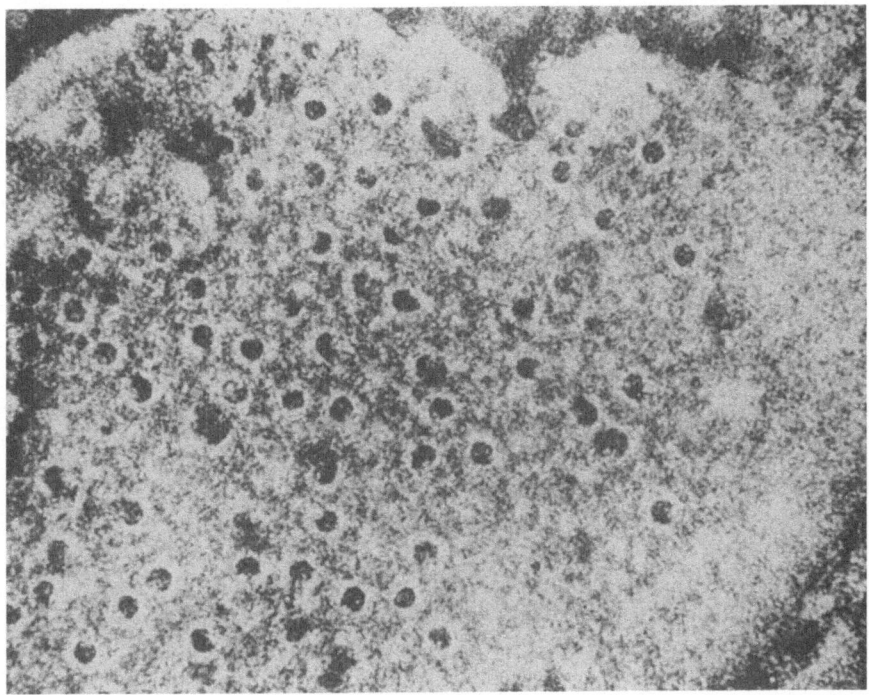

Figure 4. Complement-induced membrane lesions. Electron micrograph ($\times$ 250 000) of negatively stained *Shigella shigae* which had been treated with specific antibody and complement. The characteristic 'holes' measure about 100 Å in diameter. (Photograph by Dr. R.R. Dourmashkin.)

Complement and immune complexes

Many clinical and pathological manifestations of infectious disease result not from direct toxicity of the microorganism or its products but from hypersensitivity reactions caused by the specific allergic response of the host to microbial products (which may or may not have inherent toxic properties). One common and important group of such hypersensitivity reactions is those caused by the formation and tissue

Figure 3. Effect of complement as an opsonin. A suspension of *Salmonella typhimurium* was incubated with fresh normal human serum (as a source of complement), or with the same serum in EDTA (to inhibit complement fixation). The bacteria were then washed before being incubated at 37° with washed whole human blood. Whilst the control bacteria remained free (a) and were not ingested, the complement-treated organisms were rapidly phagocytosed and appeared (b) within the cytoplasm of polymorphs.

Table 3. Immune complex pathogenesis in microbial disease

Local formation of complexes

Allergic bronchopulmonary aspergillosis
Pulmonary lesions after respiratory syncytial virus, measles immunization
Filariasis leading to elephantiasis

Localization of complexes from the circulation

Nephropathy	post-streptococcal SBE quartan malaria
Cutaneous vasculitis	streptococci Candida M. leprae (erythema nodosum leprosum)
Polyarteritis	hepatitis B
Chronic angiitis	Trypanosomiasis

---

deposition of immune complexes between microbial antigens and humoral antibodies. Some selected examples are listed in Table 3. The factors underlying the occurrence and severity of lesions caused by immune complexes are complicated and poorly understood. In some diseases microbial characteristics are responsible for immune complex formation in all cases. On the other hand in situations where only a proportion of patients at risk suffer the immune complex lesions, for

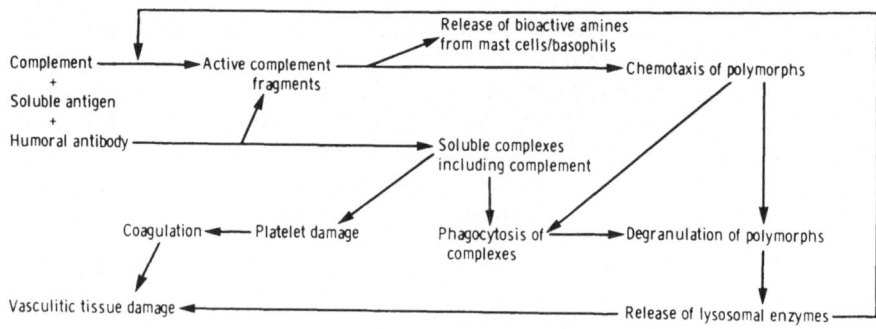

Figure 5. Type III Arthus-type (immune complex) hypersensitivity

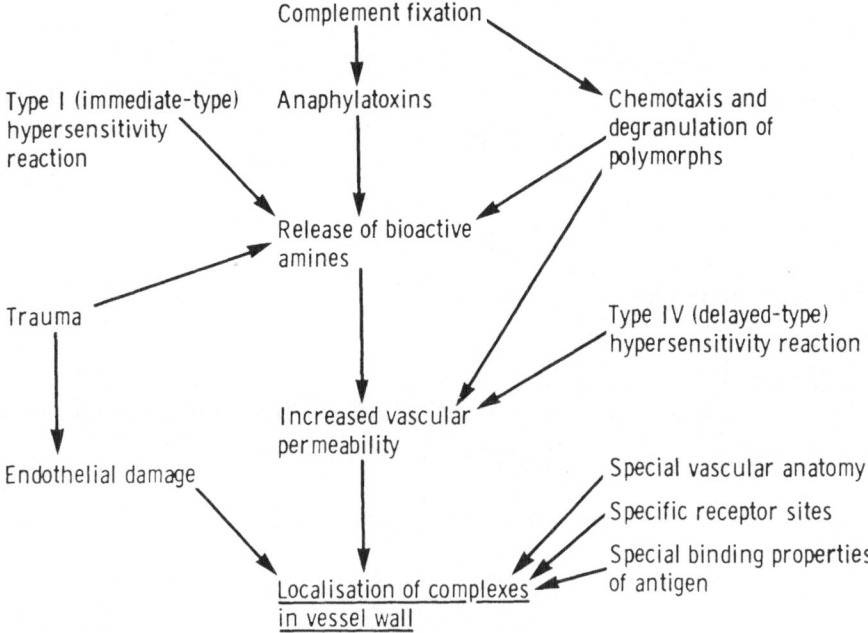

Figure 6. Localization of toxic complexes. Modified from Coombs, Gordon-Smith and Lachmann [31]

example post-streptococcal glomerulonephritis, host factors are important. Clinical and experimental observations suggest that the complement system plays a significant role in the pathogenesis of tissue damage by immune complexes [28]. Some of the mechanisms by which complement activation by immune complexes may contribute to tissue damage are illustrated in Figure 5. This sort of hypersensitivity reaction is predominantly located in blood-vessel walls and complement also plays a part in promoting the localization of toxic immune complexes at this site (Figure 6).

Until recently attention was exclusively focused on complement activation by immune complexes as a major mechanism by which they caused inflammation and tissue damage. However it has now been shown that complement not only fixes on immune complexes and promotes their adherence to cells with complement receptors, [29] but can also release them from cell surfaces (Figure 7) [29]. This complement-dependent release activity [29] results from the dissolution by complement of insoluble aggregates of antigen and antibody (Figure 8) [29]. Complement therefore seems to have a central role in modulating the *in vivo* behaviour of immune complexes, determining their size, solubility and capacity to adhere to (and therefore be taken up by or to stimulate) phagocytic and lymphoid cells. It is possible that partial, relative or even transient complement deficiencies might

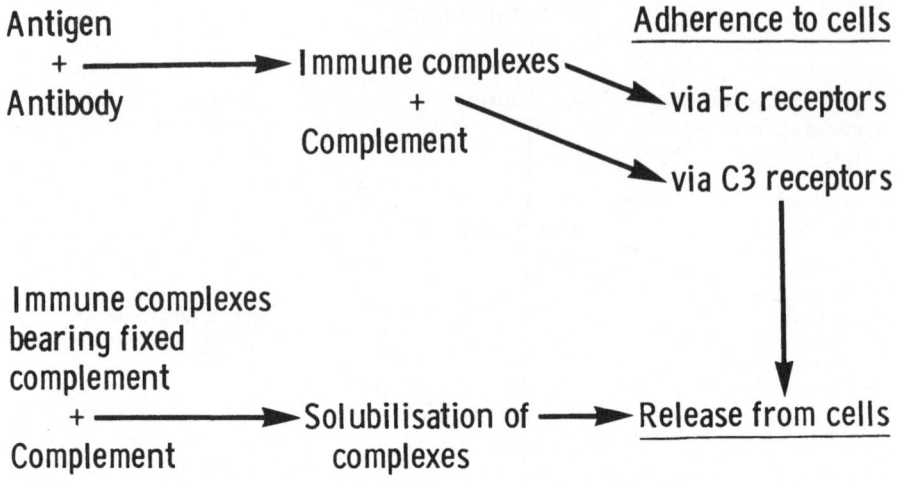

Figure 7. Complement-dependent adherence and release activity

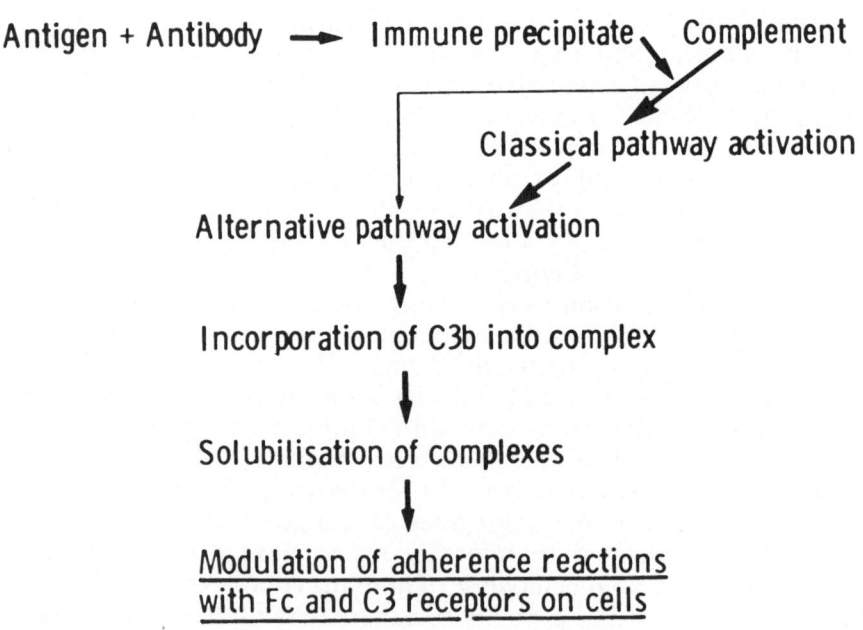

Figure 8. Solubilization of immune complexes by complement

determine whether and to what extent a patient with infectious disease suffers from complications attributable to immune complexes. This concept may provide an explanation for the otherwise perplexing observation that patients with genetic deficiency of the early complement components C1, C4 or C2 have an abnormally high incidence of inflammatory diseases of the type associated with immune-complex formation [27].

Intravascular complement activation

Severe shock with hypovolaemia, hypotension and often disseminated intravascular coagulation may occur in a number of serious infections. Clinical and experimental studies indicate that massive intravascular complement activation may be responsible for this syndrome (Table 4). It may be initiated directly by endotoxic bacterial lipopolysaccharides without the intervention of specific antibody [30], or it may

Table 4.   Clinical states of massive intravascular complement activation

Gram-negative bacterial septicaemia
     Schwartzman phenomenon
     Waterhouse–Friderichsen syndrome

Viraemia
     Dengue haemorrhagic fever
     Yellow fever

Parasitaemia
     Malaria

result from the generation of overwhelming quantities of toxic immune complexes in the circulation [31]. Some of the possible pathogenetic pathways [6, 32] are outlined in Figure 9.

Local antibody-independent complement activation

Recent experimental work has demonstrated a series of mechanisms by which microorganisms and their products might contribute to tissue damage or invoke protective immunity independently of specific allergic responses by the host. These mechanisms involve complement

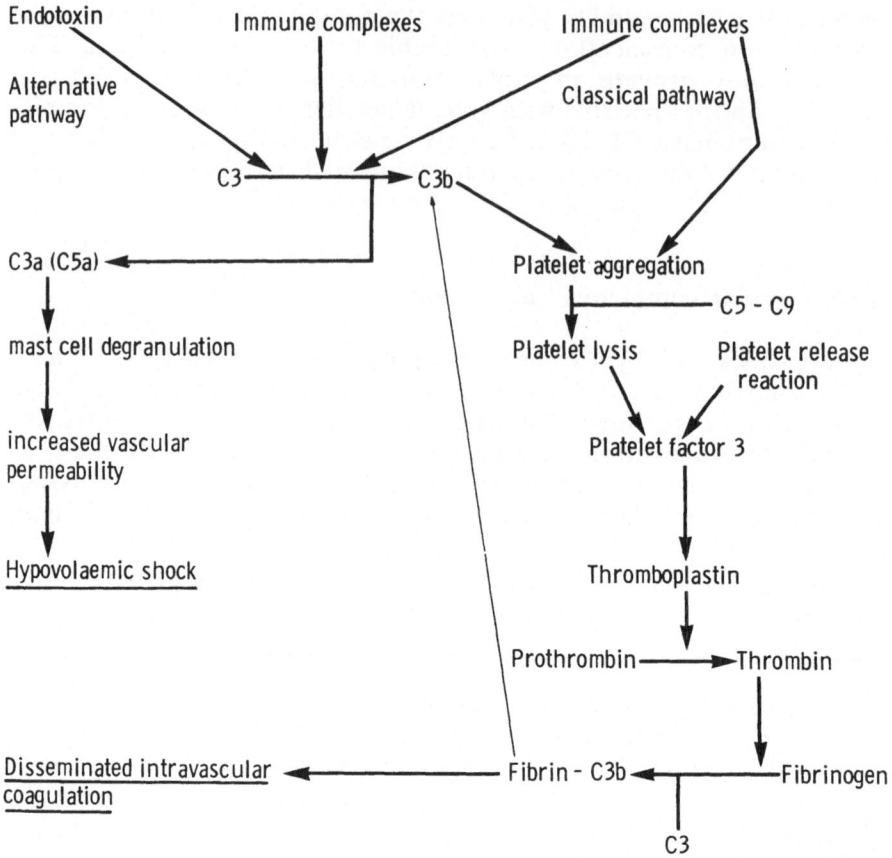

Figure 9. Coagulation and complement activation. Modified from Lachmann [6]

activation by different pathways (Table 5) and seem likely to be of clinical relevance, though this has yet to be proven. Of particular interest is the demonstration that C-reactive protein, which is an acute-phase protein produced in response to almost any tissue damage, can activate complement very efficiently [33-36]. Whether this contributes to host resistance or to microbial pathogenicity has not been determined in any particular situation.

Complement and viral infection

Although humoral antibody which neutralizes viruses can prevent them from causing infection, the major mechanism by which an

Table 5.   Local antibody-independent complement activation

Alternative pathway:	endotoxin
	bacterial polysaccharides
Classical pathway:	C-reactive protein
'Non-immunological'	leucocyte proteases
enzymes:	thrombin
	plasmin

infected host eliminates viruses from the body is by destruction of parasitized autologous cells. This can occur in an immunospecific way since viral antigens are often expressed on the surface of infected cells and can be recognized there by allergized T-lymphocytes or by antibodies. Direct killing by effector T-cells is clearly most important in the common acute viral diseases since patients with severe antibody deficiency but intact T-cells handle these normally. However, antibody-coated virus-infected target cells can also be killed by non-allergized lymphocytes or by complement fixation. In contrast, the action of antibody alone in the absence of an accessory cytotoxic effector system can merely strip viral antigens off the cell surface, leaving the cell still infected but apparently healthy and protected from destruction by the usual defences [37]. If this process were to occur *in vivo* it might form the basis for chronic asymptomatic or recurrent viral infections. The potential importance of the complement system in this immunological modulation of the consequences of virus infection results from the fact that specific antibody-dependent complement-mediated lysis of cells expressing viral antigens on their surface seems to occur via the alternative pathway [37]. This pathway is more susceptible than the classical pathway to transient or local deficiencies since it functions effectively only at or near normal plasma concentrations [4]. The efficiency of cell lysis depends on the quantity of complement available as well as the ability of the cell membrane to accept complement, the quantities of antigen expressed and antibody available and the capacity of the cell to repair membrane damage [37].

Another aspect of the interaction between complement and viruses concerns the effects of human serum on RNA tumour viruses [38]. A number of these pathogens, including Moloney, Rauscher, AKR and feline leukaemia viruses as well as Moloney and simian sarcoma viruses, are lysed by normal human complement in the absence of any specific antibody [38]. Activation takes place by the classical pathway (Figure 9), via Clq fixation, and this phenomenon may explain the failure to detect agents of this sort in human neoplastic tissues [38].

93

Summary

1. Complement activation to the stage of C3 is a mechanism of central importance in immunity, particularly with regard to invasive bacterial infection.

2. Complement plays an important part in many common aspects of microbial pathogenesis which depend upon immune-complex formation or activation of the alternative pathway.

3. Complement function may be significant in the immunological modulation of viral infection.

References

1. Colten, H.R., and Einstein, L.P. (1976) Complement metabolism: Cellular and humoral regulation. *Transplant. Rev.* **32**, 3.
2. Jersild, C., Rubinstein, P., and Day, N.K. (1976) The HLA system and inherited deficiencies of the complement system. *Transplant. Rev.* **32**, 43.
3. Shreffler, D.C. (1976) The S region of the mouse major histocompatibility complex (H-2): Genetic variation and functional role in complement system. *Transplant. Rev.* **32**, 140.
4. Müller-Eberhard, H.J. (1976) The serum complement system. In *Textbook of immunopathology*, Vol. 1, p. 45, eds. P.A. Miescher and H.J. Müller-Eberhard, 2nd edn. Grune and Stratton, New York.
5. Fearon, D.T., Daha, M.R., Weiler, J.M., and Austen, K.F. (1976) The natural modulation of the amplification phase of complement activation. *Transplant. Rev.* **32**, 12.
6. Lachmann, P.J. (1975) Complement. In *Clinical aspects of immunology*, p. 323, eds. P.G.H. Gell, R.R.A. Coombs, and P.J. Lachmann, 3rd edn. Blackwell Scientific Publications, Oxford.
7. Gewurz, H., Shin, H.S., and Mergenhagen, S.E. (1968) Interactions of the complement system with endotoxin lipopolysaccharides: Consumption of each of the six terminal complement components. *J. exp. Med.* **128**, 1049.
8. Sandberg, A.L., Osler, A.G., Shin, H.S., and Oliveira, B. (1970) The biologic activities of guinea-pig antibodies. II. Modes of complement interaction with $\bar{\gamma}1$ and $\bar{\gamma}2$ immunoglobulins. *J. Immunol.* **104**, 329.
9. Lachmann, P.J., and Nicol, P.A.E. (1973) The reaction mechanism of the alternative pathway or the C3 feedback pathway of complement fixation. *Lancet* **i**, 465.
10. Zimmerman, T.S. (1976) The coagulation mechanism and the inflammatory response. In *Textbook of immunopathology*, Vol. 1, p. 95, eds. P.A. Miescher and H.J. Müller-Eberhard, 2nd edn. Grune and Stratton, New York.
11. Lay, W.H., and Nussenzweig, V. (1968) Receptors for complement on leucocytes. *J. exp. Med.* **128**, 991.
12. Papamichail, M., Gutierrez, C., Embling, P., Johnson, P., Holborow, E.J., and Pepys, M.B. (1975) Complement dependence of localization of aggregated IgG in germinal centres. *Scand. J. Immunol.* **4**, 343.
13. Pepys, M.B. (1972) Role of complement in induction of the allergic response. *Nature New Biol.* **237**, 157.
14. Pepys, M.B. (1976) Role of complement in the induction of immunological responses. *Transplant. Rev.* **32**, 93.
15. Bokisch, V.A., Müller-Eberhard, H.J., and Cochrane, C.G. (1969) Isolation of a fragment (C3a) of the third component of human complement containing anaphylatoxin and chemotactic activity and description of an anaphylatoxin inactivator of human serum. *J. exp. Med.* **129**, 1109.

16. Shin, H.S., Synderman, R., Friedman, E., Mellors, A., and Mayer, M.M. (1968) Chemotactic and anaphylatoxic fragment cleaved from the fifth component of guinea-pig complement. *Science, N.Y.* **162**, 361.
17. Synderman, R., Phillips, J.K., and Mergenhagen, S.E. (1971) Biological activity of complement *in vivo*. Role of C5 in the accumulation of polymorphonuclear leucocytes in inflammatory exudates. *J. exp. Med.* **134**, 1131.
18. Ward, P.A., Cochrane, C.G., and Müller-Eberhard, H.J. (1966) Further studies on the chemotactic factors of complement and its formation *in vivo*. *Immunology* **11**, 141.
19. Huber, H., Polley, M.J., Linscott, W.D., Fudenberg, H.H., and Müller-Eberhard, H.J. (1968) Human monocytes: distinct receptor sites for the third component of complement and for immunoglobulin G. *Science, N.Y.* **162**, 1281.
20. Mantovani, B., Rabinovitch, M., and Nussenzweig, V.J. (1972) Phagocytosis of immune complexes by macrophages: different roles of the macrophage receptor sites for complement (C3) and for immunoglobulin. *J. exp. Med.* **135**, 780.
21. Bianco, C., Griffin, F.M., and Silverstein, S.C. (1975) Studies on the macrophage complement receptor: alteration of receptor function upon macrophage activation. *J. exp. Med.* **141**, 1278.
22. Mantovani, B. (1975) Different roles of IgG and complement receptors in phagocytosis by polymorphonuclear leucocytes. *J. Immunol.* **115**, 15.
23. Ehlenberger, A.G., and Nussenzweig, V. (1975) Synergy between receptors for Fc and C3 in the induction of phagocytosis by human monocytes and neutrophils. *Fed. Proc.* **34**, 854.
24. Scribner, D.J., and Fahrney, D. (1976) Neutrophil receptors for IgG and complement: their roles in the attachment and ingestion phases of phagocytosis. *J. Immunol.* **116**, 892.
25. Bianco, C., Eden, A., and Cohn, Z.A. (1976) Complement and macrophage activation. *J. Immunol.* **116**, 1728.
26. Schorlemmer, H.U., and Allison, A.C. (1976) Effects of activated complement components on enzyme secretion by macrophages. *Immunology* **31**, 781.
27. Lachmann, P.J. (1976) Clinical effects of complement deficiency. In *Advanced medicine* **12**, p. 43, ed. D.K. Peters. Pitman Medical Publishing Co. Ltd., Tunbridge Wells.
28. Cochrane, C.G., and Dixon, F.J. (1976) Antigen–antibody complex induced disease. In *Textbook of immunopathology*, Vol. 1, p. 137, eds. P.A. Miescher and H.J. Müller-Eberhard, 2nd edn. Grune and Stratton, New York.
29. Takahashi, M., Czop, J., Ferreira, A., and Nussenzweig, V. (1976) Mechanism of solubilization of immune aggregates by complement. Implications for immunopathology. *Transplant. Rev.* **32**, 121.
30. Brown, D.L., and Lachmann, P.J. (1973) Massive complement activation: The interactions of complement and the extrinsic blood coagulation system in the production of disseminated intravascular coagulation. *J. Immunol.* **111**, 298.
31. Coombs, R.R.A., Gordon Smith, C.E., and Lachmann, P.J. (1975) The allergic reactions as factors determining and influencing microbial pathogenicity. In *Clinical aspects of immunology*, p. 987, eds. P.G.H. Gell, R.R.A. Coombs and P.J. Lachmann, 3rd edn. Blackwell Scientific Publications, Oxford.
32. Brown, D.L. (1974) Complement and coagulation. In *Progress in immunology* II, Vol. 1, p. 191, eds. L. Brent and J. Holborow. North-Holland, Amsterdam and Oxford.
33. Kaplan, M.H., and Volanakis, J.E. (1974) Interaction of C-reactive protein complexes with the complement system. Consumption of human complement associated with the reaction of C-reactive protein with pneumococcal C-polysaccharide and with the choline phosphatides, lecithin and sphingomyelin. *J. Immunol.* **112**, 2135.
34. Siegel, J., Rent, R., and Gewurz, H. (1974) Interactions of C-reactive protein with

the complement system. I. Protamine-induced consumption of complement in acute phase sera. *J. exp. Med.* **140**, 631.

35. Siegel, J., Osmand, A.P., Wilson, M.F., and Gewurz, H. (1975) Interaction of C-reactive protein with the complement system. II. C-reactive protein-mediated consumption of complement by poly-1-lysine polymers and other polycations. *J. exp. Med.* **142**, 709.

36. Osmand, A.P., Mortensen, R.F., Siegel, J., and Gewurz, H. (1975) Interactions of C-reactive protein with the complement system. III. Complement-dependent passive hemolysis initiated by CRP. *J. exp. Med.* **142**, 1065.

37. Oldstone, M.B.A., Perrin, L.H., Tishon, A., Cooper, N.R., Lampert, P.W., and Joseph, B.S. (1976) Immunology and immunopathology of persistent virus infections. In *Advanced medicine* **12**, p. 32, ed. D.K. Peters. Pitman Medical Publishing Co. Ltd., Tunbridge Wells.

38. Cooper, N.R., Welsh, R.M., Jensen, F., and Oldstone, M.B.A. (1976) Complement-dependent lysis of RNA tumor viruses. *J. Immunol.* **116**, 1730.

Discussion

Belyavin: Is the measles rash mediated by an allergic mechanism?

Dr. Pepys: There is evidence that the rash of measles is not a direct effect of the virus itself, but is due to delayed, T-cell mediated, hypersensitivity to viral antigens. Children with congenital or acquired deficiency of T-cell function do not manifest delayed hypersensitivity. Measles infection in such individuals results in giant cell pneumonitis, presumably as a result of the failure of allergised T-cells to eliminate virus infected cells, and there is no rash.

De Louvois: How much variation is there in complement activity during life and between one individual and another?

Dr. Pepys: Complement functional activities and the levels of individual complement proteins as antigens vary within a normal range in healthy subjects. Variation outside both upper and lower limits of the normal range may occur in minor and major illnesses and may be transient or sustained (see ref. 6 above). This supports the idea that abnormality of complement function might occur at a critical phase of viral infection and affect the course of disease.

Dr. Rice: I am sure that a lot of people will have observed the effect in inactivated serum titration of occasionally meeting precipitates which have dissolved on standing: this I assume to be a complement effect and must be due to a thermostable fraction. Could you please elaborate?

Dr. Pepys: Antigen–antibody precipitates can dissolve under some circumstances in either antigen or antibody excess. This is the most probable explanation of your observation in decomplemented serum, although if heat inactivation of the complement system had been incomplete then the complement-dependent solubilization process might possibly be involved. The complement solubilization process described in ref. 29 above requires participation of both thermolabile and thermostable components.

7

Recent advances in the laboratory diagnosis of enteric virus infections

T.H. FLEWETT

Abstract

Several viruses causing infections of the gastrointestinal tract, unknown until recent years, can be detected rapidly by direct electron microscopy of faeces from patients (and from some animals also). A rapid tissue culture technique is available; its most important application is for rotaviruses. Immune electron microscopy has been of great service in detecting some of these viruses and in elucidating their serological identities.

Introduction

Nowadays there is a great emphasis on rapid diagnosis. Clinicians, and especially the younger consultants, press to know what is afflicting their patients, at least before the patients get better and go home, or die. Although this attitude is laudable, instant diagnosis is not always possible—especially in virus diseases. I do not go as far as a distinguished neuropathologist, who held that impatience on the part of clinicians for laboratory results was a sign of emotional immaturity. Nevertheless, one must take note of anxiety to know the whole truth, and try to assuage it.

Laboratory diagnosis

Virus infections can be diagnosed in three ways:
1. By detecting virus particles
   (i) by direct electron microscopy in faeces, or throat secretions, or tissue from biopsies.
   (ii) by demonstrating virus-specific proteins, which can be done by immunofluorescence or by other means.
2. By isolating and identifying viruses in tissue cultures or experimental animals, from swabs or tissues or secretions.
3. By demonstrating the appearance, during the course of disease, of antibodies to a particular virus.

The last method, though valuable for epidemiological survey work, does not yield a quick answer and is, in any case, unpopular both with children and those who have to extract blood from them.

Detection of rotaviruses

Identification by microscopy

From the point of view of viruses that parasitize cells of the gut mucosa it is fortunate that, owing to the villous expansion of the lining epithelium into the lumen, an enormous area of susceptible cells is available for the replication of viruses hardy enough to survive passage through the stomach acid. These viruses, therefore, can multiply greatly and so are shed into the lumen and hence into the faeces in enormous numbers from the infected small bowel. They may then be detected by direct electron microscopy, or by a complement fixation test, or by immune-electro-osmophoresis. For electron microscopy viruses must be morphologically recognizable, or 'labelled' in some way; and they must be numerous. For one virus particle to be present on a 70-μm grid square, dried down from a layer of liquid 0.1 mm thick, on statistical grounds 10^6 particles/ml of liquid are required, even if none is lost in the course of preparation. At a magnification of 20 000-fold, finding one virus particle on a 70-μm square is like looking for a 20-mm diameter disc on a tennis court. Given a systematic search, one can find it, but it takes time and diligence. If the virus is large and unmistakably recognizable, the diagnosis is easily made. But small and nondescript viruses can only be identified if labelled in some way, usually by being clumped by specific antiserum.

The method for electron microscopy is simple. One makes a suspension of faeces in saline or distilled water, about 20% by volume. Centrifugation at 7000 rev/min for 15 min in an angle-head rotor separates most of the undigested fat as well as the bacteria. The virus-containing liquid between the floating fat and the bacterial pellet is taken and centrifuged—50 000 rev/min for 1 hour to bring down even the smallest viruses. This virus pellet is taken up into a few drops of distilled water and mounted for electron microscopy using negative staining by methods already published [1, 2].

The interpretation is not usually difficult, if rotaviruses are present in appreciable numbers. Their structure is quite characteristic (Figure 1),

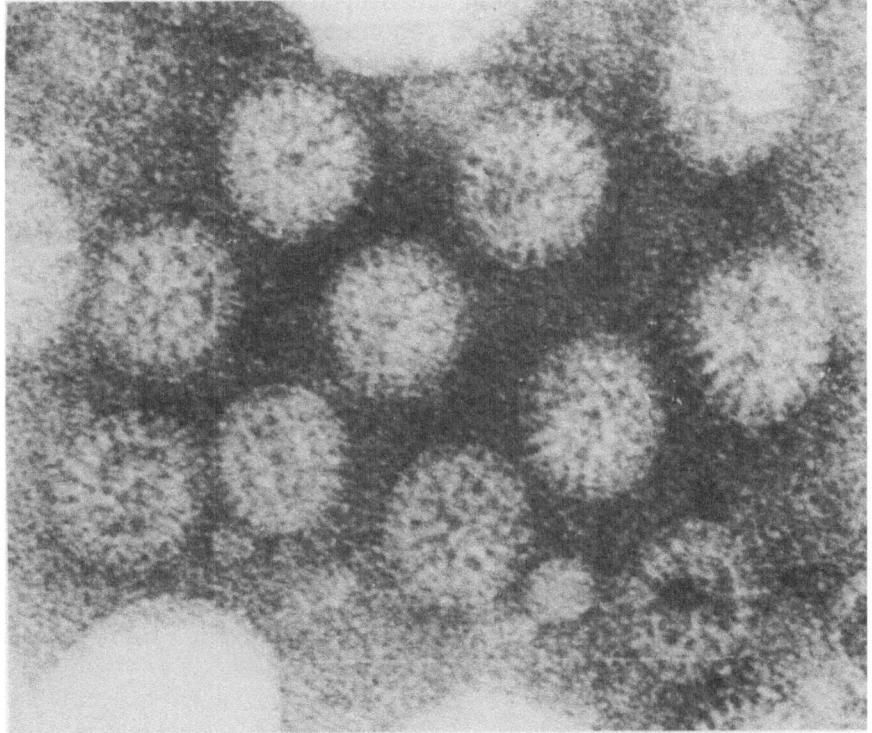

Figure 1. Rotaviruses in faeces. Usually the preparation is 'cleaner' than this, but they are clearly recognizable even though they are surrounded by debris and probably some enteric antibody. Phosphotungstate: × 296 000.

and even a single virus particle can be identified upon inspection, and its identity can be confirmed by studying a micrograph; even a single damaged particle can often be detected and identified.

Virus particles are usually plentiful, in which case it is not even necessary to centrifuge the specimen. If a suspension of faeces is merely touched to the grid, after partial drying, washing, and negative staining as described above, virus particles can be seen and identified in most specimens. Almeida (personal communication) claims 4½ minutes as the minimum time to establish a positive diagnosis. We have not timed our own procedure but agree that it is very rapid for positive diagnosis, although naturally negative specimens take longer.

Serological identification

Every practical medical microbiologist is familiar with the Widal reaction. A drop of serum from a patient convalescent from a rotavirus infection is added to a uniform, well dispersed suspension of rotavirus particles and incubated for 1–2 hours at 37° C or overnight at 4° C. The virus–antibody complexes can be centrifuged at about 15 000 rev/min for 15 min and the pellet, when mounted using negative staining, reveals aggregates of the virus. At high magnification a fuzz of antibody molecules can be seen attached to the virus particles, joining them together (Figure 2). Unfortunately, it is very difficult to establish

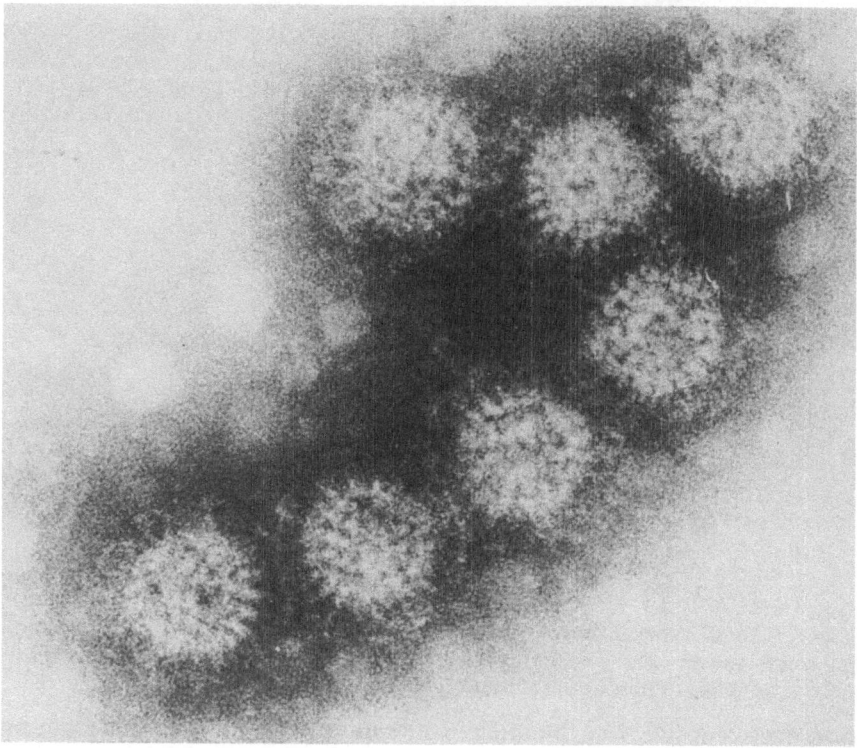

Figure 2. Rotaviruses reacted with early convalescent serum. They are surrounded by a fuzz of antibody molecules. The thicker strands are probably IgM. Phosphotungstate: × 296 000.

a titration end-point by this method. However, identification of doubtful virus particles is possible. Immune electron microscopy did, however, help to establish that the human and calf rotaviruses were closely serologically related, but not identical; and to show that this group of viruses possess a serologically similar antigen in common in the inner capsid layer [3]. Schoub *et al.* [4] have recently demonstrated a similar one-way cross-reaction between the human and monkey rotaviruses.

Cultivation of the human rotavirus in tissue culture is still very difficult, and it cannot yet be sustained indefinitely in serial subculture (see below). But the calf rotavirus has been established in serial subculture in calf kidney monolayer tissue cultures, and infected cells can be used to detect antibodies in sera from patients (Figure 3).

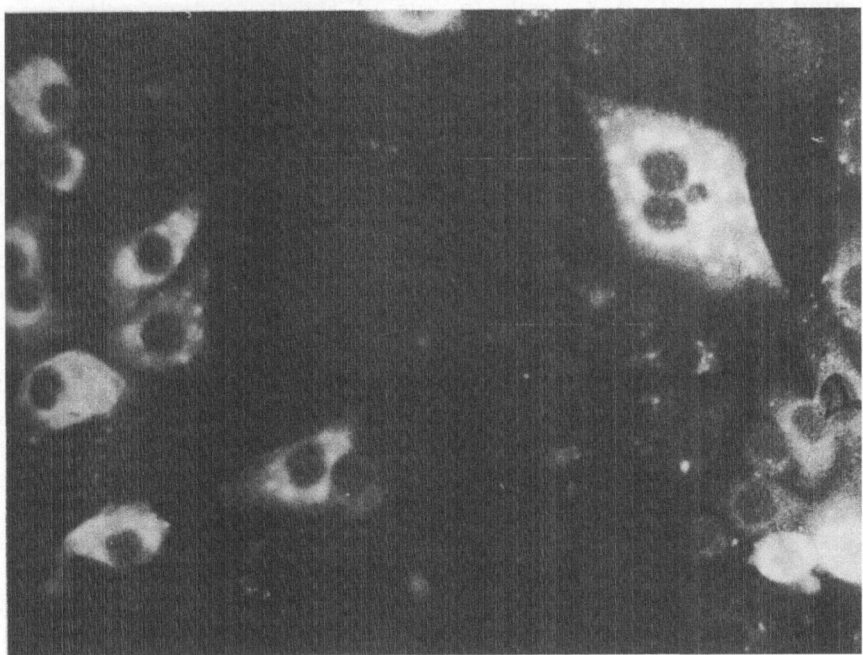

Figure 3. LLC MK$_2$ cells infected with rotavirus 18 hr previously. Virus protein occurs in granules of various sizes throughout the cytoplasm. Immunofluorescence: × 500.

Because of the strong common antigen possessed by this group of viruses, cells infected by any one of them can be used to detect antibodies to any of the others, using an immunofluorescent reaction of the ordinary 'sandwich' kind. Antibodies appear early in the course of infection, at first being mainly in the IgM class. These can be detected as early as three days after the onset of the disease and titration end-points can be determined fairly well. This technique can be used to detect antibodies appearing in the course of infection, but is mainly useful for detecting those who have, or have not, had a rotavirus infection at some time. Antibodies detectable by immuno-fluorescence persist for many years, perhaps for life.

Diagnosis by isolation in tissue culture

The methods described above are expensive and time-consuming. A rapid isolation method using tissue cultures is now available. The human rotaviruses in faeces occasionally will infect a tissue-culture cell, but often culture by orthodox methods fails completely. Banatva-la *et al.* [5] showed that rotavirus infectivity for tissue cultures could be greatly increased by centrifuging the virus inoculum on a monolayer of pig kidney cells, many of which then became infected. Bryden *et al.* [6] found that LLC MK_2 cells (a line of rhesus-monkey cells) were particularly sensitive; and that the test could be performed using Microtiter plastic plates each containing 96 wells, with a monolayer of LLC MK_2 cells on the bottom of each well. After 0.1 ml of inoculum is added to each well, the plates are centrifuged at 1000 g for 1 hour and incubated for 18–24 hr; the cell sheets are fixed in chilled methanol and infected cells 'stained' by an immunofluorescent method. The method is almost as sensitive as electron microscopy and can be used to titrate the infectivity of a specimen with reasonable precision, because three or four replicate titrations of any specimen can be easily and speedily set up. Individual infected cells can be counted by light microscopy. Results can be given the day after the specimen is received. An industrious electron microscopist does well if he examines 20–40 specimens a day, bearing in mind that it is the negative specimens which are so time-consuming; isolation in tissue culture can diagnose rotavirus infection in several hundred specimens in the same time. This method can be extended to titrate antibodies. All the known rotaviruses infect LLC MK_2 cells when centrifuged in this way, and cells infected by any of them can be detected using any convenient convalescent serum as the first layer in the immunofluorescent 'sandwich'. In this way Thouless *et al.* [7] have been able to 'type-to-species' many different rotaviruses.

Other methods of detecting rotaviruses

Virus infections can also be diagnosed by finding specific virus antigen by complement fixation, immunoelectrophoresis, or immuno-fluorescence, or by finding specific haemagglutinins. Some of these methods have been used already for rotaviruses in faeces. Much complement-fixing virus antigen is excreted in faeces of children infected with rotaviruses. Faeces, however, often contain much non-specific anticomplementary activity. Fortunately this can largely be removed by extraction of faeces by 'Arcton' or 'Arklone' (I.C.I. Ltd). An equal volume of a 20% suspension of faeces and one of these compounds is shaken for one hour. Most or all of the anti-complementary activity is removed in the fluorocarbon fraction after

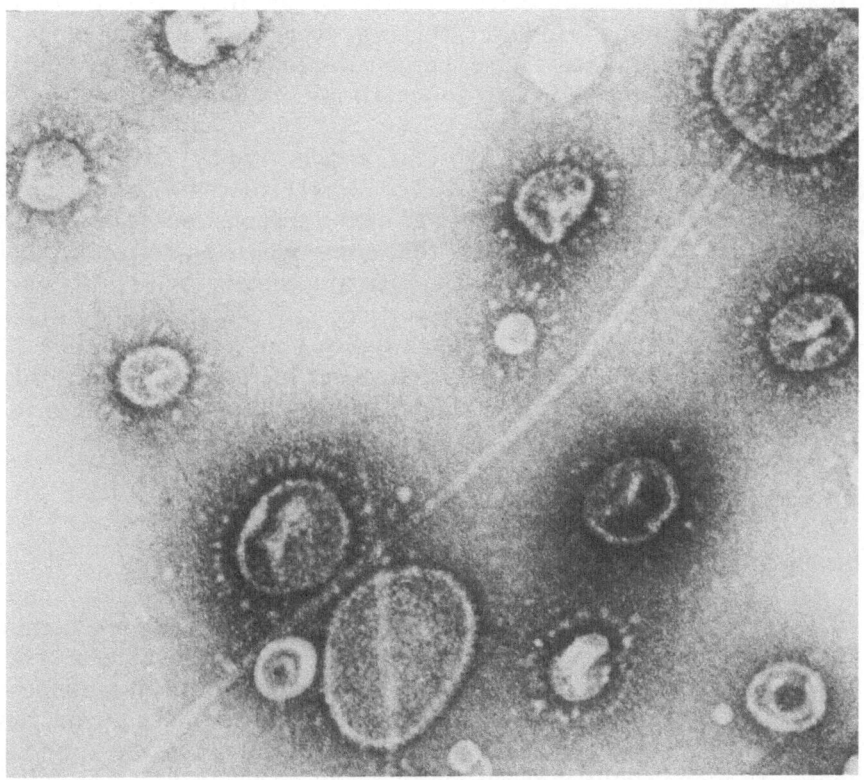

Figure 4. Coronaviruses from faeces. Uranium formate: × 296 000.

centrifuging the mixture. The remaining suspension (if the infection was a heavy one) will fix complement with a suitable antiserum, thus allowing virus antigen to be detected in the faeces. The test can be made more sensitive by concentrating the virus in the faeces by ultra-centrifugation. This method is, however, not as sensitive as electron microscopy or culture, and has still the disadvantage that one cannot always free faecal suspensions from anticomplementary activity. Another disadvantage is that guinea-pig complement may contain rotavirus group antibody so that careful controls are necessary.

Antigen may also be detected by immunoelectrophoresis. A recent report from Canada [8] shows that this method is almost as good as electron microscopy for making a positive diagnosis, provided that high-titre antibody is used. The method is the same as the immunoelectro-osmophoresis used for detection of hepatitis B surface antigen in serum, and shares its advantage in giving a positive result in one hour.

It might be predicted that antigen could be detected by spreading faeces on a slide, fixing with acetone, reacting the smear with a rotavirus antiserum, and detecting virus by 'staining' virus antigen by fluorescent antibody. However, this only works on the virus in faeces of gnotobiotic animals. Our experience is that faeces from infected children stain non-specifically, so that the method is untrustworthy for all practical clinical purposes.

Another method of detecting virus antigen, widely employed for detecting hepatitis B antigen, is to coat erythrocytes with the appropriate antibody. These, when mixed with a suspension of the antigen, are agglutinated. A difficulty is that some faecal bacteria and their flagella and fimbriae also possess haemagglutinins, and so may give non-specific positive answers. Nevertheless, it should be possible to absorb out these cross-reacting agglutinins. Thus it seems possible that haemagglutination of antibody-coated erythrocytes might afford a rapid and sensitive method for detecting rotavirus antigen in faeces.

Other diarrhoea viruses found in faeces

Adenoviruses

In all temperate countries rotavirus diarrhoea is especially prevalent in the winter months. Evidence regarding seasonal prevalence in the tropics has not been established. In the summer months it is adenoviruses rather than rotaviruses that are sometimes found as the only, or principal, virus in the faeces. Adenoviruses can often be found in faeces, though usually with difficulty, by direct electron microscopy in stools from which they have been isolated in tissue culture. In some cases of acute enteritis, both in children and occasionally in adults, adenoviruses may be found in enormous numbers by direct electron microscopy of the faeces (Figure 5). Despite their great numbers, these adenoviruses have usually not been isolated in monolayer tissue culture. This experience has been common to virologists in England, South Africa and America. Bacteriophage resembling adenoviruses in morphology are not known, and it is presumed that the observed adenoviruses multiply in the human hosts' cells. If multiplying in such large numbers, they must be assumed to be pathogenic. Homola has reported one fatal case in a child in Australia (personal communication) in which virus particles were found by electron microscopy of the small bowel at autopsy. Whitelaw *et al.* [9] have reported a similar finding in London.

Adenovirus enteritis is known in inbred Arab foals suffering from combined immunological deficiency. Takeuchi and Hashimoto [10] described adenovirus enteritis of young mice, finding abundant virus particles in the intestinal epithelial nuclei. So for adenovirus enteritis, as for the rotaviruses, analogous infections are found in animals. Although Koch's postulates have by no means been fulfilled, there is

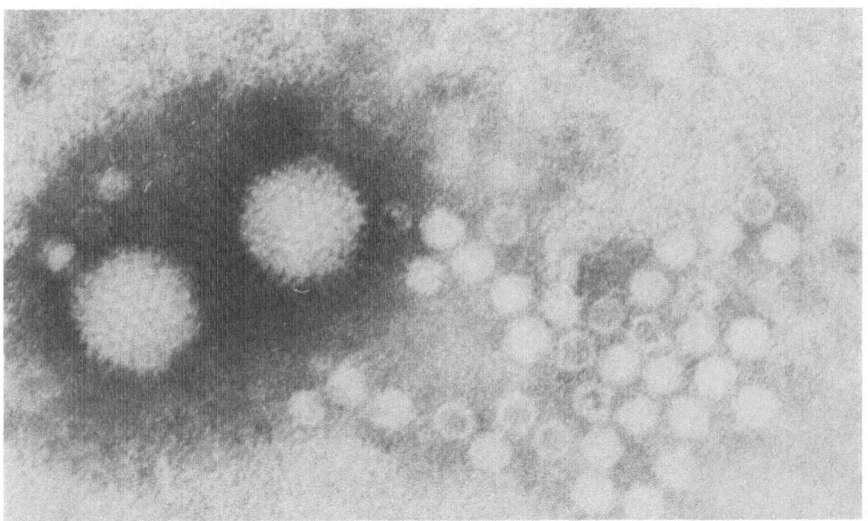

Figure 5. Adenoviruses in faeces. These are occasionally accompanied by enormous numbers of parvovirus-like particles. This preparation was not concentrated by centrifugation. Phosphotungstate: × 296 000.

thus good circumstantial evidence that adenoviruses are responsible for some cases of acute gastroenteritis in children and perhaps also in adults. Although adenoviruses have occasionally been isolated from cases of acute diarrhoea where adenovirus particles were present in great numbers, the isolations have usually been of types 1 or 2. These serotypes are often isolated from faeces of young children irrespective of disease, and may not have been the virus particles present in great abundance, but merely interlopers.

Coronaviruses

The first human respiratory pathogenic members of this group were discovered only eight years ago. The virus of transmissible gastroenteritis of piglets was found in 1970 to be a coronavirus. Bovine and canine coronaviruses infecting the intestinal tract are now known; and in 1975 Dr. Clarke's group in Bristol [11] discovered coronaviruses in faeces from young adults or teenagers in outbreaks characterized by sore throat, fever, vomiting and diarrhoea. They have succeeded in isolating these viruses in organ cultures of human embryo ileum, and subcultured them to human embryo kidney monolayer cultures. Coronaviruses sometimes occur in enormous numbers in human faeces (Figure 4). So far no method other than direct electron microscopy is available for diagnosis of human infections, though immunofluorescence techniques applied to frozen sections of bowel wall have been used for diagnosis of coronavirus enteritis in farm animals.

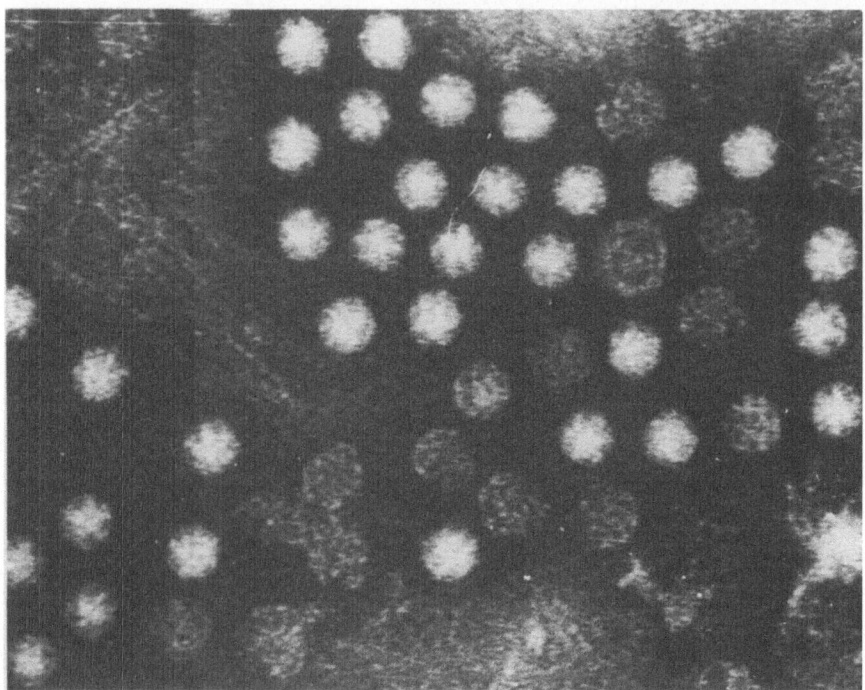

Figure 6. Astroviruses: × 300 000.

The Norwalk agent

Immune electron microscopy was used by workers in Bethesda, Maryland, to detect small (about 30 nm diameter) viruses in the faeces of volunteers who had swallowed filtrates of faeces from patients with winter vomiting disease in an outbreak in Norwalk, Conn. This virus has not so far been routinely detected in faeces in diagnostic virology laboratories.

Astroviruses

These are small viruses, about 28 nm in diameter, spherical or isometric in shape, sometimes found in faeces in large numbers (Figure 6). When negatively stained these viruses show upon their surface a 5- or 6-pointed star structure. They also show up, at low magnification, in rather more contrast than most small viruses, giving an appearance on the fluorescent screen of the electron microscope, of the sky at night, each virus particle a star. Hence the name 'astrovirus' proposed for these viruses by Madeley and Cosgrove.[12] Their structure is easily distinguishable from that of ordinary enteroviruses. They have been found in the faeces of young children with diarrhoea, but also frequently in faeces of healthy children. It seems likely that they are indeed pathogens. Infected convalescent children produce antibodies which agglutinate them. Bovine astroviruses are now known (Woode and Bridger (1976) personal communication).

Caliciviruses

These again have a characteristic structure, with small depressions— 'calices'—upon their surfaces. Like astroviruses, they have frequently been found in healthy children, and their importance as pathogens has not been firmly established. A strain causing diarrhoea in kittens is known, so that there is a good animal model. Caliciviruses from cats, pigs and sea-lions have been established in tissue culture, but human strains have not yet been isolated.

References

1. Flewett, T.H., Bryden, A.S., and Davies, H. (1974) Diagnostic electron microscopy of faeces. I. The viral flora of the faeces as seen by electron microscopy. *J. clin. Path.* 27, 603–8.
2. Flewett, T.H., and Boxall, E.H. The hunt for viruses in infections of the alimentary system: an immunoelectron-microscopical approach. *Clin. Gastroenterol.* 5, 359–85.
3. Flewett, T.H., Bryden, A.S., Davies, H., Woode, G.N., Bridger, J.C., and Derrick, J.M. (1974). Relation between viruses from acute gastroenteritis of children and new-born calves. *Lancet* ii, 61–3.
4. Schoub, B.D., Lecatsas, G., and Prozesky, O.W. (1977) Antigenic relationship between human and simian rotaviruses. *J. Med. Microbiol.* 10, 1–6.
5. Banatvala, J.E., Totterdell, B., Chrystie, I.L., and Woode, G.N. (1975) *In vitro* detection of human rotaviruses. *Lancet* ii, 821.
6. Bryden, A.S., Davies, H., Thouless, M.E., and Flewett, T.H. (1977) Diagnosis of rotavirus infection by cell culture. *J. Med. Microbiol.* 10, 121–5.
7. Thouless, M.E., Bryden, A.S., Flewett, T.H., Woode, G.N., Bridger, J.C., Snodgrass, D.R., and Herring, J.A. (1977) Serological relationships between rotaviruses from different species as studied by complement fixation and neutralization. *Archs Virol.* 53.
8. Middleton, P.J., Petric, M., Hewitt, C.M., Szymanski, and Tam, J.S. (1976) Counter-immunoelectro-osmophoresis for the detection of infantile gastroenteritis virus (orbi-group) antigen and antibody. *J. clin. Path.* 29, 191–7.
9. Whitelaw, A., Davies, H., Parry, J. (1977) Electron microscopy of fatal adenovirus gastroenteritis. *Lancet* i, 361.

10. Takeuchi, A., and Hashimoto, K. (1976) Electron microscope study of experimental enteric adenovirus infection in mice. *Infect. Immun.* **13**, 569-80.
11. Caul, E.O., Paver, W.K., and Clarke, S.K.R. (1975) Coronavirus particles in faeces from patients with gastroenteritis. *Lancet* i, 1192.
12. Madeley, C.R., and Cosgrove, B.P. (1975) Viruses in infantile gastroenteritis. *Lancet* ii, 124.

Discussion

Prof. Mimms: We are getting used to very sophisticated explanations of the pathophysiology of diarrhoea. Could you comment on that matter for the rotaviruses. Do you think that loss of the disaccharidase-containing cells is a factor?

Dr. Flewett: Yes, I am sure it is. Fatal infections are comparatively rare in the human and if the human child comes to an autopsy it is usually a day or two later and the post-mortem histology is not worth much. Evidence from infected piglets and calves indicates that it is the cells that make the disaccharidases which these viruses attack. There is about 70 g per litre of lactose in human milk. Cow milk is 'humanized' by adding sugar. This amount of lactose alone is just about isotonic. Disaccharides are not absorbed but monosaccharides are. If a large amount of disaccharide is ingested when the virus has destroyed the disaccharidase-producing cells, the disaccharides are not hydrolysed. So there is an extra osmotic load going down the small bowel preventing absorption of water from it. Under normal circumstances when disaccharides are hydrolysed the glucose moiety acts as a sort of pump which also transports water. But worse is to come: all this lactose then goes down unsplit into the large bowel where there are plenty of lactose splitting organisms; but these do not just split lactose into glucose and galactose. One molecule of lactose will be split into about six molecules of short-chain acids and this exerts an enormous osmotic effect. You might as well give the child a dose of Epsom salts! The corollary to this is that, if you treat these virus infections simply by cutting off the disaccharide intake, you get an almost miraculous improvement. The patient stops having diarrhoea: this has been observed in medical and veterinary practice.

I was taught when I was a student that you should treat a child with acute gastroenteritis by stopping its milk supply and give it albumin water instead. Nowadays, they have a much fancier solution of electrolytes which they use. But the same effect applies.

Dr. Damjanovic: Do you find classic enteroviruses by your technique?

Dr. Flewett: You can if there are a lot of them there. Last year we were absolutely flooded with Echo 19 infection but only in one third of these could we find virus particles by direct electron microscopy in the faeces. If we mixed the faecal supernates with an Echo 19 antiserum we could get nice aggregates. Even in poliomyelitis it is unusual to get as many as 10^6 infective particles per g of faeces.

8

The role of *Chlamydia trachomatis* in female genital infections and in conjunctivitis of the newborn

DEREK HOBSON and ELISABETH REES

Abstract

Chlamydia trachomatis is now frequently found in association with non-gonococcal urethritis in men, and it can be isolated from the cervical secretions of a proportion of their sexual contacts. Until recently, there have been difficulties in establishing the diagnosis of chlamydial infection with precision. Thus there is only circumstantial evidence that the presence of this organism in the female genital tract has any pathological significance for the woman herself or for any infants born whilst her infection is active.

This chapter discusses the development of simplified and improved rapid methods of laboratory diagnosis of *C. trachomatis* infections. These can now give results of a sensitivity and reproducibility similar to those used in the investigation of gonorrhoea. One such method has been applied by us in Liverpool for the past three years to the investigation of contacts of men with non-gonococcal urethritis, and to other groups. The presence of chlamydial infection has been correlated

with the clinical findings in the uterine cervix, and it is apparent that infection during pregnancy can be associated with puerperal pyrexia, as well as with the development of conjunctivitis in the offspring.
There are strong indications for effective antibiotic treatment, with clinical and laboratory follow-up, of all women with chlamydial infection of the cervix.

Background

'Nothing is new. We walk where others went.' R. Herrick, 1648.

Historical introduction

Over the past few years there has been a marked and progressive increase in forms of sexually-transmitted disease (STD) which can cause clinical and epidemiological confusion with gonorrhoea, but which have no apparent bacterial or viral aetiology. In fact, non-gonococcal urethritis is now almost twice as prevalent as gonorrhoea in males in England. In 1975 alone there were 69 826 new male cases of non-gonococcal urethritis as against 37 377 new male cases of gonorrhoea. On epidemiological grounds, and by analogy with gonorrhoea, it was to be suspected that the female consorts of males with non-gonococcal urethritis might be persistent but probably silent reservoirs of the infective agent or agents.
The apparently new perspective in the clinical microbiology of non-gonococcal urethritis and related conditions is the recent recognition that:

1. Non-gonococcal urethritis often fails to respond satisfactorily to regimes of antimicrobial therapy which are effective cures for gonorrhoea or for mycoplasmal infections [1].

2. Approximately 50% of males with non-gonococcal urethritis are now found to have *Chlamydia trachomatis* infections of the urethra.

3. Approximately 30% of the female sexual partners of men with non-gonococcal urethritis have chlamydial infection of the cervix.

4. Infants born to some infected women develop conjunctivitis from which *C. trachomatis* can be isolated.

This triad of urethritis in the male, cervicitis in his partner and ophthalmia neonatorum in their offspring has obvious resemblances to gonorrhoea.
There is nothing new in this situation, except perhaps in scale and in the relative ease of diagnosis. Almost 70 years ago Halberstaedter and von Prowazek [2] in Germany showed that no bacterial cause could be found for some cases of ophthalmia neonatorum but scrapings of conjunctival cells from these infants revealed intracytoplasmic inclu-

sions very similar to those they had previously described in patients with hyperendemic tropical trachoma [3]. Moreover, cell scrapings from the cervix of the mother and from the urethra of the father (some of whom had clinical signs or symptoms of urethritis) often contained similar intracellular inclusions [4]. Even though these early workers were not able to isolate the presumed infectious agent, they showed that the direct inoculation of cell scrapings from the eye or genital tract of patients into the conjunctiva of monkeys resulted in gross infection with scarring and blindness, closely similar to the picture of trachoma. It took another half-century for their results to be verified by laboratory procedures. In 1957, T'ang and his colleagues [5] isolated the first strains of *C. trachomatis* from classical cases of hyperendemic trachoma in China, by inoculating conjunctival scrapings into the yolk sac of chick embryos. Shortly afterwards, T'ang's method was applied to the investigation of non-bacterial ophthalmia neonatorum in London. A trachoma-like agent was isolated from the eye of an affected infant and from the cervix of her mother. When laboratory cultures of this strain were rubbed on to the conjunctiva of baboons, a severe ophthalmia developed, and scrapings showed conjunctival cells containing intracytoplasmic inclusions [6].

Throughout the 1960s, further investigations using the chick-embryo yolk-sac technique showed that indigenous males with clinically-active non-gonococcal urethritis in London and urethral infection with such trachoma-inclusion conjunctivitis agents [7, 8]. However, these egg-inoculation techniques proved too cumbersome, slow, insensitive and prone to cross-contamination to be readily applied to large-scale diagnostic and epidemiological studies, and they have now been almost entirely superseded by tissue-culture isolation procedures.

Trachoma-inclusion conjunctivitis agents isolated from cases of genital infection and conjunctivitis in Europe or the USA are now known to differ serologically from *C. trachomatis* strains from cases of classical trachoma in tropical countries [9, 10] but, all have very similar biological properties. They can readily be differentiated from the chlamydial agent of lymphogranuloma venereum and from *C. psittaci*, which is widely distributed as a pathogen in the animal kingdom, where it can cause ocular and genital infections as well as the well-known generalized infection of parrots and other birds.

It is now clear that chlamydiae are not true viruses, and have many of the characteristics of bacteria, e.g. the possession of both DNA and RNA, as well as cell walls containing muramic acid and innate enzyme systems which render them susceptible to many antibacterial chemotherapeutic agents [11]. However, chlamydiae are obligate intracellular parasites, which depend upon the host mammalian cell for their energy sources, such as adenosine triphosphate, and hence their isolation in the laboratory demands technical procedures similar to those used in the diagnosis of viral infections.

Culture of *C. trachomatis*

It has been known for many years that *C. psittaci* and lymphogranuloma venereum agent can be grown successfully in a variety of conventional replicating mammalian cells in tissue culture, where they produce intracytoplasmic inclusions filled with elementary bodies, similar to those in the cells of naturally infected animals [12]. However, the growth of *C. trachomatis* in tissue culture has presented several practical problems which have limited the general application of tissue-culture methods in the routine investigation of the role of these agents in STD. In particular many of the cell lines used for diagnostic virology are not highly susceptible to *C. trachomatis* infection or require special techniques to make them so. The widely used McCoy cell line, originally selected because it was thought to be a line of human synovial cells, is now known to be a mouse fibroblastic tumour-cell line. Because of their neoplastic nature, McCoy cells divide quickly and repeatedly with no contact inhibition of growth, to produce dense sheets of packed cells with little cytoplasm, and nutrients in the growth medium are rapidly exhausted. Hence, the growth of chlamydiae is likely to be impaired and difficult to detect unless special precautions are taken to provide suitably enriched media and to slow down or

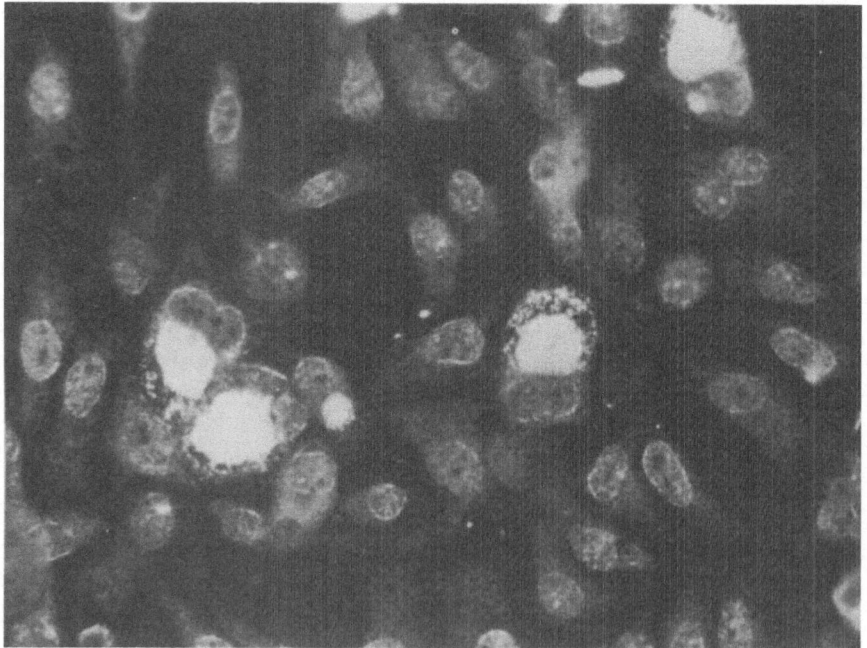

Figure 1(a) L (light-ground microscopy)

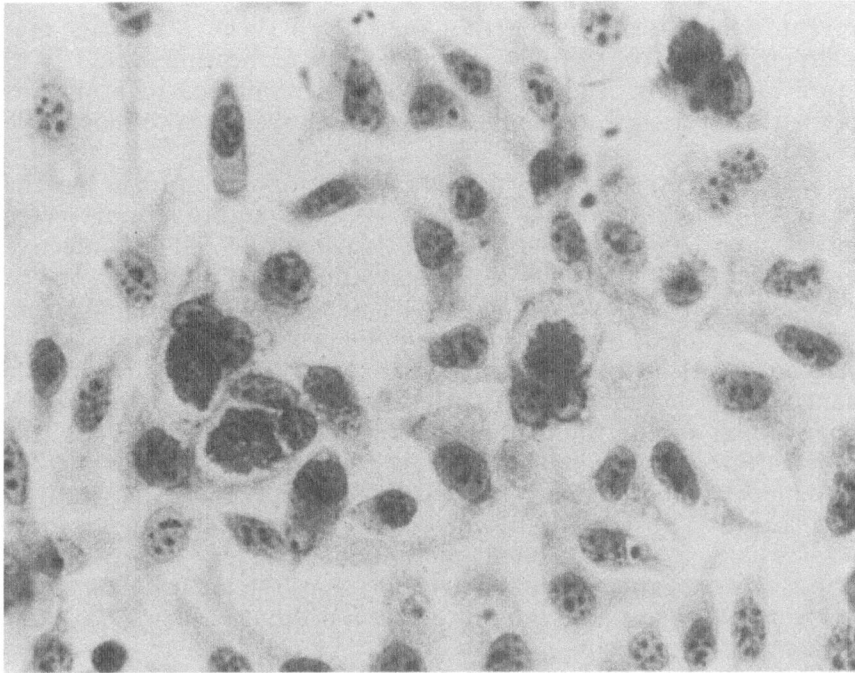

Above: **Figure 1(a) D (dark-ground microscopy)**
Below: **Figure 1(b)**

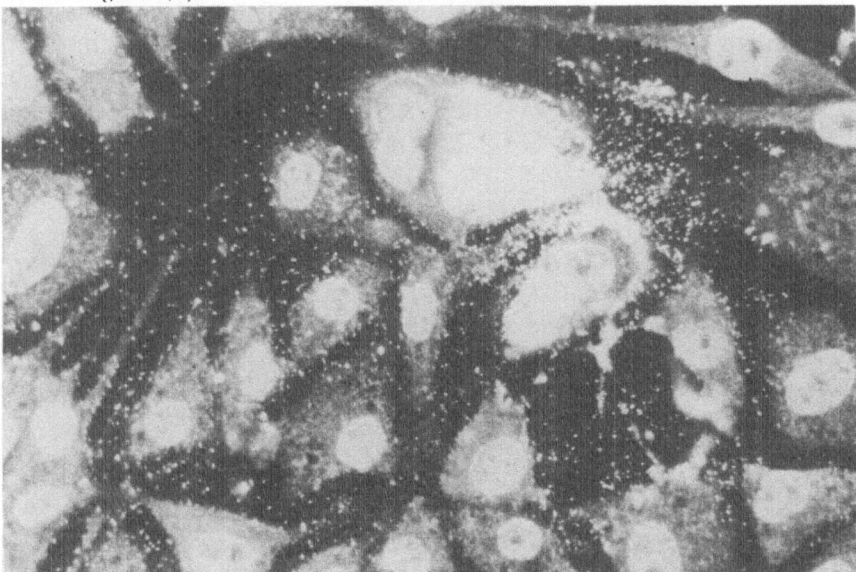

Figure 1. Giemsa-stained McCoy cell monolayers showing intracytoplasmic inclusions of *C. trachomatis* **(× 400).**
(a) after incubation 37° 48 hr: L = light-ground microscopy. D = dark-ground microscopy, showing innate fluoresence of inclusions.
(b) after incubation 37° 72 hr, showing bursting inclusions

113

prevent cell division. Irradiation of the cell sheet [13], or its pre-
treatment with deoxyuridine [14] or other anti-replicating agents [15, 16]
before inoculation of clinical specimens is often used to bring this
about. However such methods add extra complications to diagnostic
procedures.

The main problem, whatever the nature of the tissue culture, is that the
uptake of *C. trachomatis* by the cells in tissue-culture monolayers is
inefficient. Effective contact between tissue-culture cell and infective
particles can best be achieved by centrifuging the inoculum on the
tissue-culture monolayer at 2500 *g* for 1 hr at 33° C before incubation.
A further problem is that *C. trachomatis* usually gives only a single
cycle of growth in tissue culture. There is no cumulative cytopathic
change, and the number of intracellular inclusions detectable is
proportional to the number of input infective particles. Thus, the
tissue-culture cell monolayer, which is grown on flying coverslips for
convenience, needs to be removed, fixed and Giemsa-stained after
48–72 hrs and inspected for inclusions under × 400 microscopy,
preferentially by dark ground illumination (Figure 1). Beyond this
period, false negative results may occur, since the inclusions mature,
rupture the host cell and fall off the glass without inducing daughter
inclusions in fresh cells.

Laboratory procedures for the isolation of *C. trachomatis* from
patients with genital infections are labour-intensive and time-consuming. In our view, these methods are still not feasible for large-scale
open-ended routine diagnosis in STD clinical practice and accordingly
we have largely restricted their use to an epidemiological survey in one
particular STD clinic in Liverpool Royal Infirmary.

Objectives of our study

Our main aims were to determine (a) how frequently *C. trachomatis*
was found in various categories of women attending the clinic, and (b)
whether this agent behaved as a primary pathogen, producing definite
signs and symptoms in its own right, or whether it should be regarded
only as a secondary opportunistic invader in genital disorders of other
aetiology, or indeed even as part of the normal genital flora.

Methods

In Liverpool, normal replicating cultures of McCoy cells have been
used successfully. We have already described [17] the procedures which
are summarized in Figure 2.

It was first necessary to confirm that the laboratory isolation procedures were sufficiently sensitive and reproducible for long-continued
epidemiological studies. Details of these standardization tests have

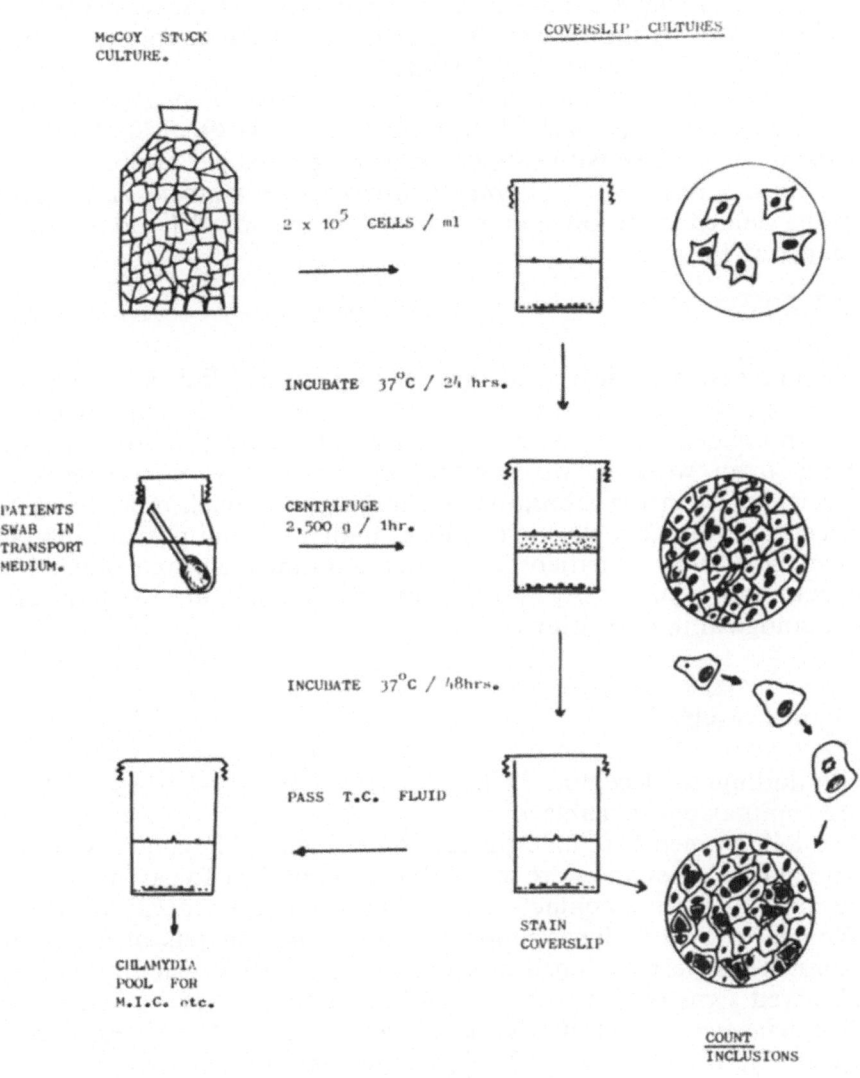

Figure 2. The diagnostic procedure for isolating *C. trachomatis* **in tissue culture** [17]. The liquid growth medium in the 1-oz screw-cap bottles consists of 2 ml of medium 199 + 10% foetal calf serum

been described elsewhere [17, 18]. Briefly, quantitative counts of the number of inclusions produced by clinical specimens provide the most simple running check on the efficiency of the laboratory procedure:

1. When a single culture of *C. trachomatis* was inoculated on 48 replicate McCoy monolayers 95% of the inclusion counts fell within 23% of the mean value over the whole series.

2. When cervical swabs from 153 *C. trachomatis*-positive women were repeated 7 days later, before treatment, 141 (92.5%) of women were again positive with similar inclusion counts per swab.

3. In a series of 175 *C. trachomatis*-positive women, 72% of the swabs yielded inclusion counts of over 100 and only 8% had inclusion counts of 10 or lower.

Interpretation

The practical significance of such findings to the clinician is that the precision of diagnosis of *C. trachomatis* infections can approach that of gonorrhoea. Small inescapable variations in the prescribed procedures from week to week, either in the quality or transport of specimens or in the laboratory techniques, are much more likely to affect the average inclusion counts of patients found positive than to alter the number of patients so scored. Routine inclusion counts thus provide an inbuilt early warning of any slippage in long-term epidemiological investigations.

Clinical results

Our findings to December 1976, with cervical swabs from 1421 women, are summarized in Table 1.

The 949 women first investigated, in a single STD clinic, were not consecutive cases and were selected because of the clinical findings, or because they were contacts of men with non-gonococcal urethritis. Women known to have gonorrhoea or to be contacts of men with gonorrhoea were excluded in order to reduce the possibility that the observed signs or symptoms might be due to gonorrhoea and not to *C. trachomatis* infection. Cervical swabs from 32.9% of these women yielded *C. trachomatis* on McCoy monolayer cultures.

In a gynaecological out-patients clinic, 40/171 women (23.4%) were found to have chlamydial infection of the cervix. These were selected cases; most had been referred from other gynaecological clinics for further investigation of vaginitis, cervicitis or pelvic infection, and the high incidence rate was undoubtedly biassed by the fact that 21 mothers of infants with chlamydial conjunctivitis were examined and found to be *C. trachomatis*-positive in this clinic.

In contrast to the findings in these clinics, *C. trachomatis* was not

Table 1. **The incidence of genital infections with** *C. trachomatis* **in women in Liverpool 1974-76**

Category of women	Total	Chlamydia Positive	% Positive
STD clinic	949	312	32.9
Gynae. out-patients	171	40	23.4
Infertility clinic	31	0	0
NGU contacts — consecutive	203	71	35
Known gonorrhoea — consecutive	67	36	53.7
Totals	1421	459	32.3

isolated from cervical swabs of any of 31 women on their first attendance at an Infertility Clinic in the same hospital. To further clarify the picture, we examined two groups of consecutive patients, unselected except in that the first group consisted of 203 patients referred as contacts of men with non-gonococcal urethritis, and the second group of 67 patients with gonorrhoea diagnosed by smear and/or culture within the last few days, but untreated.

The first group contained both primary (source) contacts and secondary contacts, and most of the latter were wives or regular partners of affected men; 35% of them were found to have chlamydial infection, but, as is the case with contacts of gonorrhoea, many of the *C. trachomatis*-infected women had no symptoms or clinical signs.

The highest incidence of chlamydial infection of the cervix was found in women with gonorrhoea; 53.7% of them were found to have concurrent infection with *C. trachomatis*. This high incidence has been confirmed recently in a larger group of women in Liverpool (Davies, Rees, Byng and Hobson—unpublished). A similar high isolation rate (63%) has been found in Bristol [19], but in a London clinic only 33% of women with gonorrhoea were found to have concurrent *C. trachomatis* infection [20]. This difference may reflect a lower overall level of chlamydial infection in the community in areas where routine treatment of non-gonococcal urethritis contacts, on epidemiological grounds, has been the policy.

A high incidence of concurrent gonorrhoea and *C. trachomatis* infection in sexually active women is a finding with potentially serious implications. In many STD clinics there are no special facilities for isolating chlamydia; hence, the patients' signs and symptoms and her positive contact history may well be attributed solely to her gonorrhoea. This infection can usually be confirmed rapidly, and will commonly be treated only by single-dose regimes of penicillin which, until recently, have usually been curative. However, penicillin is not fully effective against chlamydia *in vitro*, and frequently fails to eradicate chlamydial genital infections [21 22 23]. Thus there is a distinct risk that these women will return to the community from the STD clinic as persistent unsuspected reservoirs of one of the two infections they had on arrival. In our experience, chlamydial infections of the cervix can persist for many months unless specific therapy, e.g. with tetracyclines or erythromycin, is instituted. Hence, these women may continue to spread infection to their sexual partners, and may themselves possibly develop clinical complications of their chlamydial infection, especially if they are, or become, pregnant.

Our failure to isolate *C. trachomatis* from patients in infertility clinics, in contrast with the high incidence in women in STD clinics, supports the view that the patients' life-style influences the probability of chlamydial infection. It has been suggested that this agent might be no more than a secondary invader or even part of the 'normal' microbial flora of promiscuous sexually active young women. However the high frequency of infection in these women makes it essential, in our opinion, to determine whether *C. trachomatis* behaves as a primary pathogen of the female genital tract.

Accordingly, we have correlated the laboratory and clinical findings in 254 non-gonococcal urethritis contacts. This was a selected group in which 127 chlamydia-positive women were compared with 127 chlamydia-negative cases. The frequency of infection with *Candida* species, *Trichomonas* or herpes virus was not significantly different in the two groups of women; gonococci were isolated from four of the *C. trachomatis*-positive and two of the *C. trachomatis*-negative group, after they were admitted to the series.

The results (Table 2) show a significantly raised incidence of *C. trachomatis* in women with hypertrophic (oedematous) cervical erosions and endocervical mucopus. This strongly suggests that *C. trachomatis*, like gonorrhoea, can give rise to pathological changes at the site of infection in some cases. In fact, our current observations (Davies *et al.*, Tait, Rees, Hobson and Johnson—unpublished) appear to indicate a similar incidence of pathological findings with either of the two infections.

Treatment of chlamydia-positive women with oxytetracycline, and their subsequent follow-up for periods of up to one year, have shown [24] that the cessation of detectable chlamydial infection was followed shortly by a change from mucopurulent exudate to clear or cloudy mucus in the endocervix and by a change from hypertrophic to non-pathological simple erosion; in a few cases metaplasia occurred. However, relapsed infection or re-infection of these women was associated with a return of the previous clinical signs.

Table 2. Clinical signs in the cervix in 254 selected contacts of men with non-gonococcal urethritis (*C. trachomatis* was isolated from 127 cases)

		Chlamydia		%
		Positive	Negative	Positive
	No erosion	28	61	31.5
Cervical	Simple erosion	53	51	50.9
appearance*	Hypertrophic erosion	40	6	86.9
	Chronic cervicitis	5	9	
	Clear mucus	31	76	28.9
Cervical	Cloudy mucus	28	36	43.7
contents+	Mucoid or mucopus	64	11	85.3
	Blood	4	3	

* One chlamydia-positive patient not recorded.
+ One chlamydia-negative patient not recorded.

Examination of the eyes of newborn babies with chlamydia-positive conjunctivitis, and the genital tracts of their mothers, gives further evidence that genital strains of *C. trachomatis* fulfil Koch's postulates and can be regarded as primary pathogens. We have investigated 103 infants, most of whom were referred to us because they had conjunctivitis for which no bacterial cause had been found, or because they had failed to respond within a few days to routine treatment with eye drops or ointment of neomycin or chloramphenicol. These infants are thus a selected group, and not a representative sample of all the infantile 'sticky eye' seen in maternity units. In 33 of these infants *C. trachomatis* was isolated from eye swabs. Details of their clinical history, bacteriology and treatment are described elsewhere [25]. In 27 cases *C. trachomatis* was the sole pathogen, but in three babies there was concurrent infection with *N. gonorrhoeae*, in two others with *Staph. aureus* and with herpes simplex virus in one case. Chlamydial infection was frequently associated with purulent exudate and with oedema of the lids and mucosa. These signs quickly disappeared after treatment with tetracycline eye ointment. However, prolonged observation was necessary after the 4–6-week period of treatment. Re-occurrence of symptoms with re-isolation of chlamydia have been found in inadequately-treated infants, and we are at present assessing a combined schedule of systemic erythromycin with a shortened course of topical tetracycline.

In none of this series was the baby born of a previously-diagnosed but untreated mother, i.e. the baby was the prime indicator of infection in the family. Investigation of 31 mothers of chlamydia-positive babies showed that 21 had chlamydial infection of the cervix, but seven of the culture-negative mothers had already been started on courses of broad-spectrum antibiotics because of post-partum pyrexia or infected lochia. In total, 19 of the mothers of chlamydia-positive infants developed evidence of puerperal infection and pelvic inflammatory disease was found in 11 women. In 8 out of 9 cases investigated serologically, antibody against the group antigen of chlamydia (detectable by complement fixation with commercial *C. psittaci* antigen) was found in high titre (greater than 1/40). In four of these where serial serum samples were obtained, there was a four-fold or greater rise in titre. Thus, it seems possible that *C. trachomatis* can not only behave as a pathogen capable of causing cervical lesions, but can under certain circumstances spread more widely in the genital tract and pelvic tissues to give a more generalized infection. In fact, *C. trachomatis* has recently been isolated directly from the affected tube of two patients with salpingitis [26].

This suggestion of ascending infection of the female genital tract with *C. trachomatis* led us to postulate that, in pregnant women with chlamydial infection of the cervix associated with oedema and purulent discharge, spread of infection to the membranes overlying the os might occur and lead to premature rupture. This has not yet been confirmed but indirect evidence in support of this hypothesis has been obtained. In the series of 103 babies with sticky eye, where the basis of referral by the paediatrician was the same throughout, 14/33 (42.4%) *C. trachomatis*-positive babies had been delivered prematurely as against 9/58 (15.8%) *C. trachomatis*-negative infants. The development of chlamydia-positive conjunctivitis in one pre-term infant in the series who was born by caesarian section after premature rupture of membranes supports this hypothesis of ascending chlamydial infection.

Conclusions and implications

Non-gonococcal infections associated with infections by chlamydia resembling the causative organism of hyperendemic trachoma are not a new phenomenon. From the beginning of this century it has been clearly recognized that men with chlamydial urethritis can infect or be infected by their sexual partners and that babies born of infected mothers can develop ophthalmia neonatorum with a very similar clinical picture to that caused by gonorrhoea.

Recent evidence suggests that these conditions have become increasingly common. This correlates with the continuous rise in the incidence of gonorrhoea throughout the last two decades despite the ease of recognition and treatment of that disease. This increase has been attributed to greater promiscuity and a decreased use of barrier contraceptives. In fact the ability, until recently, to cure gonorrhoea quickly has been one of the major factors in highlighting other forms of STD such as mycoplasmal and chlamydial infections, which do not respond so readily to antibiotic therapy. Some of the apparent recent increase in chlamydial STD may, however, be the result of an increasing awareness of its existence, coupled with the development of simplified laboratory diagnostic procedures which are now becoming little more complex than those routinely employed in the diagnosis of common virus infections.

Much of the emphasis of recent investigation of chlamydial infection has been on the infected male, who usually develops a brisk clinically-obvious urethritis. As with gonorrhoea, the female partner is likely to develop a much less clinically manifest but persistent genital infection. The results we have presented and discussed above suggest that the female is not a reservoir of *C. trachomatis* merely of nuisance value to the sexually active male. Therefore consorts of men with non-gonococcal urethritis deserve full investigation and treatment not merely on epidemiological grounds, but because of hazards to their own health. Hypertrophic cervical erosions appear to occur frequently in association with the infection and may be the starting point of further spread in the genital tract, as in gonorrhoea, and of puerperal pelvic inflammatory disease, and might thus affect the woman's subsequent fertility. The remote possibility exists that this combination of a chronic intracellular infection with hypertrophic changes in the cervix may be yet another co-factor in the aetiology of carcinoma of the cervix, as postulated for the herpesviruses.

Most of the cervical infections with *C. trachomatis* we have seen occurred in women aged 17–25 years, at the peak child-bearing age, and are often clinically inapparent. Thus it is to be expected that infants born to infected women are at risk. The development of ophthalmia neonatorum, as seen in our investigations, can approach the severity of that caused by the gonococcus. This has long been recognized, but recently it has been suggested [27] that *C. trachomatis* infection of the neonate can also result in a clinically distinctive respiratory syndrome.

There are now increasingly widespread and probably justifiable requests from gynaecologists, as well as venereologists, for nationwide routine facilities for the diagnosis of chlamydial infections, as for gonorrhoea, to form a rational basis for antibiotic therapy and for epidemiological control of non-gonococcal genital infection. An informed decision can best be made by a rapid expansion of large scale epidemiological studies. It is particularly important to determine the frequency, duration, relapse rate and complications of chlamydial infections of the female genital tract over the country as a whole, and in populations other than those largely self-selected women who choose to attend STD clinics in the larger cities.

Note

The investigations reported in this Chapter were supported by a project grant from the Medical Research Council.

References

1. Bowie, W.R., Alexander, E.R., Floyd, J.F., Holmes, J., Miller, Y., and Holmes, K.K. (1976) Differential response of chlamydial and ureaplasma-associated urethritis to sulphafurazole (sulfisoxazole) and aminocyclitols. *Lancet* i, 1276–8.
2. Halberstaedter, L., and von Prowazek, S. (1909) Ueber chlamydozoen befunde bei Blennorrhöe neonatorum non gonorrhoica. *Berlin klin. Wochschr.* **46**, 1839.
3. Halberstaedter, L., and von Prowazek, S. (1907) Zur Aetiologie des Trachoms. *Deutsche med. Wochschr.* **33**, 1285–7.
4. Lindner, K. (1910) Zur Ätiologie der gonokokkenfreien Urethritis. *Wien. klin. Wochschr.* **23**, 283.
5. Tang, F.F., Chang, C.L., Huang, Y.T., and Wang, K.C. (1957) Studies on the etiology of trachoma with special reference to isolation of the virus in chick embryo. *Chin. med. J.* **75**, 429–47.
6. Jones, B.R., Collier, L.H., and Smith, C.H. Isolation of virus from inclusion blennorrhoea. *Lancet* i, 902–5.
7. Dunlop, E.M.C., Al-Husseini, M.K., Garland, J.A., Treharne, J.D., Harper, I.A., and Jones, B.R. (1965) Infection of urethra by TRIC agent in men presenting because of 'non-specific' urethritis. *Lancet* i, 1125–8.
8. Dunlop, E.M.C., Freedman, A., Garland, J.A., Harper, I.A., Jones, B.R., Race, J.W., Du Toit, M.S., and Treharne, J.D. (1967) Infection by Bedsoniae and the possibility of spurious isolation. 2 Genital infection, disease of the eye, Reiter's disease. *Am. J. Ophthalmol.* **63**, 1073–81.
9. Treharne, J.D., Dines, R.J., and Darougar, S. (1977) Serological responses to chlamydial ocular and genital infections in the UK and Middle East. In *Non-gonococcal urethritis and related oculo-genital infections*, eds. Hobson, D., and Holmes, K.K. American Society for Microbiology, Washington D.C., 249–58.
10. Kuo, C.-C., Caldwell, H.D., Wang, S.-P., and Grayston, J.T. (1977) Antigens of chlamydia trachomatis. In *Non-gonococcal urethritis and related oculo-genital infections*, eds. Hobson, D., and Holmes, K.K. American Society for Microbiology, Washington D.C., 176–85.
11. Becker, Y. (1974) The Agent of Trachoma. Recent studies on the biology, biochemistry and immunology of a prokaryotic obligate parasite of eukaryocytes. *Monographs in Virology*, vol. 7. S. Karger, Basel.
12. Bland, J.O.W., and Canti, R.G. (1935) Growth and development of psittacosis virus in tissue culture. *J. Path. Bact.* **40**, 231–41.
13. Gordon, F.B., Dressler, H.R., Quan, A.L., McQuilkin, W.T., and Thomas, J.T. (1972) Effect of ionizing radiation on susceptibility of McCoy cell cultures to *C. trachomatis*. *Appl. Microbiol.* **23**, 123–9.
14. Wentworth, B.B., and Alexander, E.R. (1974) Isolation of *Chlamydia trachomatis* by use of 5-iodo-2-deoxyuridine-treated cells. *Appl. Microbiol.* **27**, 912–16.
15. Sompolinsky, D., and Richmond, S. (1974) Growth of *Chlamydia trachomatis* in McCoy cells treated with cytochalasin B. *Appl. Microbiol.* **28**, 912–14.
16. Ripa, K.T., and Mårdh, P.-A. (1977) A new simplified culture technique for

Chlamydia trachomatis. In *Non-gonococcal urethritis and related oculogenital infections,* eds. Hobson, D., and Holmes, K.K. American Society for Microbiology, Washington D.C., 323–27.

17. Johnson, F.W.A., and Hobson, D. (1976) Factors affecting the sensitivity of replicating McCoy cells in the isolation and growth of chlamydia A (TRIC agents). *J. Hyg., Camb.* **76**, 441–51.
18. Johnson, F.W.A., Hobson, D., Rees, E., and Tait, I.A. (1977) Quantitative aspects of the growth of *Chlamydia trachomatis* in diagnostic tissue culture procedures. In *Non-gonococcal urethritis and related oculo-genital infections,* eds. Hobson, D., and Holmes, K.K. American Society for Microbiology, Washington D.C., 309–13.
19. Hilton, A.L., Richmond, S.J., Milne, J.D., Hindley, F., and Clarke, S.K.R. (1974) Chlamydia A in the female genital tract. *Br. J. vener. Dis.* **50**, 1–10.
20. Oriel, J.D., Powis, P.A., Reeve, P., Miller, A., and Nicol, C.S. (1974) Chlamydial infections of the cervix. *Br. J. vener. Dis.* **50**, 11–16.
21. Johnson, F.W.A., and Hobson, D. (1977) The effect of penicillin on genital strains of *Chlamydia trachomatis* in tissue culture. *J. antimicrob. Chemother.* **3**, 49–56.
22. Hobson, D., Rees, E., Johnson, F.W.A., and Tait, I.A. (1977) The effect of penicillin on *Chlamydia trachomatis in vitro* and *in vivo.* In *Non-gonococcal urethritis and related oculo-genital infections,* eds. Hobson, D., and Holmes, K.K. American Society for Microbiology, Washington D.C., 227–29.
23. Oriel, J.D., Ridgeway, G.L., Reeve, P., Beckingham, D.C., and Owen, J. (1976) The lack of effect of ampicillin plus probenecid given for genital infections with *Neisseria gonorrhoeae* on associated infection with *Chlamydia trachomatis. J. infect. Dis.* **133**, 568–71.
24. Rees, E., Tait, I.A., Hobson, D., and Johnson, F.W.A. (1977) Chlamydia in relation to cervical infection and pelvic inflammatory disease. In *Non-gonococcal urethritis and related oculo-genital infections,* eds. Hobson, D., and Holmes, K.K. American Society for Microbiology, Washington D.C., 67–76.
25. Rees, E., Tait, I.A., Hobson, D., Byng, R.E., and Johnson, F.W.A. (1977) Neonatal conjunctivitis caused by *Neisseria gonorrhoeae* and *Chlamydia trachomatis. Br. J. vener. Dis.* **53**, 173–79.
26. Mårdh, P.-A., Ripa, T., Wang, S.-P., and Westrom, L. (1977) *Chlamydia trachomatis* as an etiological agent in acute salpingitis. In *Non-gonococcal urethritis and related oculo-genital infections,* eds. Hobson, D., and Holmes, K.K. American Society for Microbiology, Washington D.C., 77–83.
27. Beem, M.O., and Sazon, E.M. (1977) Respiratory tract colonization and a distinctive pneumonia syndrome in infants infected with *Chlamydia trachomatis. New Engl. J. Med.* **296**, 306–10.

Discussion

Prof. Brumfitt: I am very interested in the proposal that there is a relationship between neonatal conjunctivitis and prematurity.

Dr. Hobson: We've mentioned this briefly, elsewhere. There were 33 positive and 58 negative children. We looked at the age of those children. We found that 42% of the babies with chlamydia-positive conjunctivitis were premature. This compared with 15.8% of the chlamydia-negative babies who were premature. This is significant at the 5% level. Obviously something we want to follow up. We don't yet have any real idea of why this is occurring. We thought at first it was because premature infants stay in hospital longer, but this is not so. We thought perhaps this might be associated with immunological deficiency in the premature infant. I am not too happy that this is the explanation. Since we know that the chlamydial cervix can develop grosser hypertrophic erosions in late pregnancy and just after pregnancy in the premature infant: I am not too happy that this is the might be causing severe endocervicitis. The amount of pus there suggests this is possible. The chlamydia may be extending into the amniotic membrane overlying the cervix, and thus be responsible for softening the membrane, causing premature rupture, causing prematurity and infecting the emerging baby. It might be possible that some infants are infected *in utero*, not in passing through the cervix.

Mr. Slade: Has Dr. Hobson had the opportunity of investigating cases of 'sterile' pyuria? I ask this because there is a condition that clinicians label 'abacterial pyuria' which is associated with a very acute cystitis, equally in men and women. The clinical criteria which you describe in the way of oedema, mucopus, angry mucosa are fulfilled. In the past I am sure these cases were treated with antituberculous therapy. I have got a personal series of about six. I have taken biopsies of the bladder and each one responded dramatically to treatment with oxytetracycline. I am convinced that these infections were due to chlamydia.

Dr. Hobson: That is very interesting. Recently, there have been papers on experimental chlamydia infections in the guinea pig and the macaque monkey. The urethritis observed wasn't an anterior urethritis but it involved the whole length of the urethra. This often occurs in man, too. They can develop epididymitis from chlamydia. In the monkey the lesions are very much like those in the eye and the cervix and there is gross oedema and engorgement. We've only seen one chlamydia-positive woman who was referred to us with a primary complaint of dysuria rather than coming from a special clinic.

Dr. Rees: One of the difficulties associated with urinary tract infections is that by the time one sees the patient they have had a lot of antibiotic therapy. We have had one interesting case referred from the urological unit, a young woman with recurrent cystitis over a period of two or three years developed abacterial pyuria. She had not recently received antibiotics and was found on cystoscopy to have an acute urethritis—not cystitis. The gynaecologist found a hypertrophic cervix with mucopus in the endocervix. When I examined her I found mucopus and oedema of the urethra and we had an isolate of chlamydia from the urethra and the cervix which responded to tetracycline.

Dr. Hobson: It is interesting that Mr. Slade's cases responded to tetracycline. One of the guiding features for saying that chlamydia is in causal association with the type of condition we have been describing is that when chlamydia-positive urethritis or cervicitis is treated with oxytetracycline the symptoms and chlamydia go away. The presence of another underlying tetracycline-sensitive pathogen which has been missed is most unlikely because there was no response in chlamydia-negative patients who are matched for severity or duration of symptoms.

9

Microbial aspects of patients with leukaemia

A.V. HOFFBRAND

Numerous authors have pointed out that infection is assuming increasing importance as the major cause of death in patients with leukaemia and other malignant disease. This situation arises partly because of the increased use of cytotoxic drugs in combination, at high doses. When given for prolonged periods such treatment makes patients susceptible to infection because of neutropenia and immunosuppression. It is also partly because control of haemorrhage has resulted in improved survival rate, the availability of platelet concentrates and concentrates of clotting factors having improved in recent years. Much of the research into the aetiology, prevention and treatment of infection in patients with malignant disease or those with neutropenia from whatever cause, has been carried out on patients with acute myeloblastic leukaemia. This Chapter reviews some of the findings and conclusions in such patients. Major reviews of all aspects of infections in patients with haematological diseases have recently been published [1-3].

Predisposing factors

Neutropenia is the major predisposing factor to infection in patients with malignant disease [4], and this is particularly likely to occur in acute leukaemia where therapy aimed at producing a remission inevitably results in bone-marrow suppression with periods of pancytopenia. In general, therapy for myeloblastic leukaemia causes more profound bone-marrow failure than anti-lymphoblastic leukaemia therapy, since drugs selective against lymphocytes, e.g. vincristine and prednisone, have little effect against myeloid tissue. Neutrophil counts below $1.0 \times 10^9/1$ lead to increased incidence of infection and the frequency rises steeply when the count falls. More than 30 episodes of severe infection occurred per 1 000 days spent with counts less than $0.1 \times 10^9/1$ [5]. Moreover, acute myeloblastic leukaemia or acute lymphoblastic leukaemia cause a reduction in the numbers of circulating mature neutrophils and monocytes while bone-marrow reserves are also depleted. Granulocytopenia may be aggravated by transfusion of ABO incompatible red cells or of HLA mis-matched platelets, probably through deposition of immune complexes on the granulocytes which are then destroyed in the reticulo-endothelial system [6]. Susceptibility to infection because of granulocytopenia is aggravated by accompanying monocytopenia due to the disease or to the cytotoxic drug therapy. In addition, in acute myeloblastic leukaemia the neutrophils and monocytes that are produced are functionally incompetent as judged by tests of chemotaxis such as the skin-window technique, phagocytosis and of intracellular killing of bacteria. Corticosteroid therapy may also impair granulocyte function and for this reason therapy given on alternative days if possible is preferred [7].

Immune suppression due to drugs or radiotherapy also leads to increased susceptibility to infection. Cytotoxic drugs, particularly cyclophosphamide, 6-mercaptopurine (and azathioprine), methotrexate and 5-fluorouracil are especially likely to impair function of lymphocytes, particularly B-cells, while corticosteroids and radiotherapy tend to impair T-cell function [8]. Patients with chronic lymphocytic leukaemia often show impaired immunoglobulin synthesis and this may be a major factor in their susceptibility to infection particularly in the later stages of the disease. Humoral immunity is relatively well preserved in acute leukaemia.

Types of infection and causative organisms

Bacterial

In most reports, the most common infecting organisms are the Gram-negative bacilli, *Pseudomonas aeruginosa*, *Escherichia coli* and *Kleb-*

Table 1. Relative frequency of bacterial pathogens in acute leukaemia

Comparison of causes of infection in two large series (Valdiviesco, 1976, M.D. Anderson Hospital, Texas; Gaya 1975, Hammersmith Hospital, London).

Valdiviesco [9].		Gaya [2].	
Bacterial organisms causing fatal infection		Septicaemia with documented cause	%
Number of infections of known aetiology	214	Ps. aeruginosa	31
Bacterial infections (% of total)	82	E. coli	20
		Klebsiella/Enterobacter/Serratia	11
Gram-negative bacilli (% of total infections)	76	Proteus spp.	2.5
		Staph. aureus	13
% of Gram-negative bacilli		Staph. albus/Micrococcus	4
E. coli	29	Streptococci	2.5
Ps. aeruginosa	21	Clostridia	7
Klebsiella/Enterobacter/Serratia	50	Other bacteria	4
		Fungi	2.5
		Pneumocystis carinii	2.5

siella spp. (Table 1). In the United States *Serratia* and *Enterobacter* species are also common in leukaemic patients. In a recent study, 75% of patients with acute myeloblastic leukaemia died as a direct result of infection and 76% of identified bacterial infections were due to Gram-negative bacilli [9]. Most fatal infections are disseminated or pulmonary. In a minority of patients, Gram-positive cocci, such as *Staphylococcus aureus*, *Staph. epidermidis* or *Streptococcus faecalis* are responsible. Anaerobic bacteria, viruses or fungi can seldom be found to be the cause of severe infection in patients with acute myeloblastic leukaemia (see below).

The explanation for the high incidence of Gram-negative bacillary infection is related to host susceptibility and environmental factors. In the neutropenic patients, organisms not normally pathogenic may play an opportunistic role. The host's own enteric bacteria are often the source of infection. Colonization and subsequent infection by Gram-positive cocci was at one time common but this has diminished with the introduction of β-lactamase stable penicillins such as cloxacillin. On the other hand, Gram-negative bacilli seem to be relatively resistant to normally used hospital antiseptics and antibiotics. As many as 40% of acute myeloblastic leukaemia patients may become colonized with Gram-negative organisms after admission to hospital. The incidence of clinical infection following colonization seems to be particularly high in the case of *Pseudomonas aeruginosa*. Food and other commodities delivered to the patient may be sources of contamination, as well as hospital sinks, floors, hospital personnel and even flowers.

Infections in neutropenic patients tend to be severe. In a recent series, as many as 22% of episodes of septicaemia in acute myeloblastic leukaemia were caused by multiple organisms [10], often with combinations of *Ps. aeruginosa*, *E. coli* and *Staph. aureus*. The most common sources of the septicaemia have been found to be gastrointestinal ulceration, skin infections and pneumonia.

Fungal infections

Fungal are much less common than bacterial infection in leukaemia, but a significant incidence of fungal infections has been reported in the United States, but the incidence is lower in Britain. At post-mortem, an incidence of 13 to 31% of major fungal infection has been reported in four American series in which histological evidence of tissue invasion has been sought [11], although this had not been detected clinically. Other clinical studies reveal a much lower incidence of infection. For instance, among 100 children with acute lymphoblastic leukaemia treated at St. Jude's Hospital (England), only one was reported to have developed life-threatening fungal infection [12], while among 39 infectious episodes in 27 patients with acute leukaemia or advanced lymphoma studied by Rodriguez *et al.* [13], none could be definitely ascribed to fungi. Recent studies by Levine *et al.* [14] and Klastersky *et al.* [15] showed an incidence of 25% and 12% respectively of fungal infection among episodes of severe infection. However, lack of a precise definition of fungal infection and absence of tissue diagnosis in many cases makes it difficult to assess a true incidence. In Great Britain, probably less than 5% of all serious infections in acute leukaemia patients have been found to be due to fungi.

Viral infections

Certain viral infections such as those with rhinoviruses, adenoviruses and enteroviruses, are no more common in immunosuppressed patients with leukaemia than in the rest of the population. Furthermore, these patients do not suffer a more serious infection than other subjects with these organisms. On the other hand, infection with varicella-zoster, herpes simplex, cytomegalovirus, rubella and vaccinia seem to be more common in patients with haematological malignancy, and these patients tend to suffer a more severe form of the disease [16]. Nevertheless, in adult patients with acute leukaemia, serious viral infections are much less frequent than bacterial infection. In lymphomas, however, the relative frequency of viral infection is greater. For instance, it has been estimated that between 15 and 25% of patients with stage III or IV Hodgkin's disease suffer from herpes zoster infection, while a 10% incidence has been recorded in children with acute lymphoblastic leukaemia or lymphosarcoma. Herpes zoster is particularly likely to occur after irradiation.

Diagnosis of infection

Because of the low neutrophil count and impaired inflammatory response, it may be difficult to diagnose the site and type of infection. Surveillance by cultures at least once a week of urine, stool, throat, saliva, sputum, groin, axillae, vagina, etc. may suggest the nature of the organism involved. In these patients, fever is the best indication of infection and must always be taken seriously. Within hours of fever developing, swabs must be taken from the suspicious areas mentioned above. At least two blood cultures should be taken, and urine and swabs from sputum, throat and intravenous cannulae should be cultured and a chest X-ray carried out. Tests to speed diagnosis have been devised. These include the Limulus test for endotoxin and the nitroblue tetrazolium test to differentiate fever of bacterial origin (with a positive test); [67]gallium-citrate administration with subsequent organ scanning to localize infection has been recommended. Unfortunately none has been found to be sufficiently reliable to provide a basis for definite diagnosis and treatment. Even in the best hands in about 40%

of febrile episodes in acute myeloblastic leukaemia patients the cause of the fever is not diagnosed. (This applies even in those patients where the fever resolves following antibiotic therapy [17].)

Antibiotic therapy

A number of studies have confirmed the value of broad-spectrum combination antibiotic therapy in neutropenic patients with acute leukaemia who have fever, before the identity of the infecting organism and its antibiotic sensitivity is known. This approach has reduced considerably the number of early deaths from Gram-negative septicaemia. Choice of antibiotic is determined by the need to use drugs which are effective in the absence of neutrophils; for example, polymyxins are ineffective in neutropenic patients and gentamicin is less effective in neutropenic than normal patients. The lack of a single effective antibiotic has led to the use of combinations [18]. The antibiotics used must, of course, be active against Gram-negative bacilli. Frequent combinations used are carbenicillin (e.g. 5 g every 4 hours) plus gentamicin (e.g. gentamicin 1.25 mg/kg body weight every 6 hours), carbenicillin plus a cephalosporin (e.g. cephalothin 2 g every 4 hours). Some physicians use a combination of all three of these antibiotics. A recent controlled trial has suggested that amikacin, which is an aminoglycoside related to kanamycin A, is at least as effective as gentamicin and no more nephrotoxic or ototoxic, although prospective studies on vestibular function remain to be carried out on a large scale [19]. The semi-synthetic penicillins carbenicillin and ticarcillin are particularly valuable because they are active against *Ps. aeruginosa* and are equally effective in neutropenic and normal patients. However, in the high dosage needed they may impair platelet function and if this occurs it may lead to increased haemorrhage [20]. Amikacin is best reserved for infections known to be resistant to gentamicin and other aminoglycosides. Sissomicin is another aminoglycoside, related to gentamicin, which also appears to be valuable in neutropenia. Tobramycin is a new aminoglycoside which may be particularly effective against *Pseudomonas* spp. [21] or *Klebsiella* spp. [5]. Gaya *et al.* [22] found that any two of these three antibiotics were equally effective in neutropenic, immunosuppressed patients but, as others have reported [23], the combination of gentamicin and cephalothin whether alone or with carbenicillin as well, is particularly nephrotoxic and is best avoided. The response rate to these antibiotics in neutropenic patients has gradually risen over the last few years, mainly due to the earlier institution of the therapy. Improved cure rates with no increase in nephrotoxicity have also been reported when the aminoglycoside is administered by continuous infusion [24].

Antibiotic therapy is continued for at least 5 days after the temperature becomes normal. If an organism is identified after 'blind' therapy has been started, appropriate antibiotics are added and inappropriate antibiotics discontinued as soon as possible. Blood levels should be monitored since renal function is often impaired in these patients, and a blood bactericidal titre above 1:16 maintained for the organism isolated, if possible. If the temperature fails to fall after several days of antibiotic therapy (with, if possible, granulocyte transfusions), it may be necessary to discontinue all therapy and perform new cultures in an attempt to identify the infection. Viral and fungal infections should always be considered when antibacterial chemotherapy fails.

Where the site of infection is known, it may be advisable to alter the initial anti-fever regimen. For instance, although the documented incidence of Gram-negative anaerobic infection is low in these patients, the true incidence may be higher and where bowel lesions or lesions of the ano-rectal region are present, metronidazole should be added to the initial therapy.

Prophylaxis

The measures taken vary widely from one centre to another. In some special centres, the patient is decontaminated as far as possible by oral non-absorbable antibiotics, anti-fungal and antiseptic lozenges, douches and creams to orifices, and if a bacterial pathogen is isolated, systemic antibiotic therapy. A typical oral regime is 'FRACON' (framycetin, colistin and nystatin). Other antibiotics used include a combination of paromomycin sulphate, polymyxin B sulphate and vancomycin hydrochloride or of gentamicin sulphate and vancomycin hydrochloride. Alternative antifungal agents include amphotericin B or candicidin (polyene antibiotics). In some units, these antibiotics and antifungal agents are used topically but others prefer to use only non-antibiotic antiseptic agents locally (e.g. phisohex or iodinated soap) to reduce emergence of organisms resistant to antibiotics and hypersensitivity to them.

The patient is nursed in isolation with reverse-barrier nursing, sterile food, and possibly filtered air-flow or even a life-island. Life-islands are not generally used because of the difficulty in nursing and the psychological and physical problems for the patient living in a confined space for a prolonged period. Laminar air-flow rooms with sterilization of all objects including food entering the room, with all personnel entering wearing sterile caps, masks, gowns, gloves and boots, are more acceptable, and provide an equally effective protective environment with settle plates showing only about 6% pathogens and 60% sterile when the patient is receiving oral antibiotic prophylaxis [25, 26]. Problems exist in sterilizing the surfaces and particularly sinks in these rooms. Elimination of the patient's bacteria from stool, throat, ear, nose, vagina and skin is about 70 to 95% effective, and of fungi up to 80% effective. Any persisting organisms are usually not conventional pathogens. The groin and perianal region are skin areas from which it is particularly difficult to eliminate pathogens while some patients acquire new strains of bacteria and fungi, particularly in the throat, stools and skin, as a result of the prophylactic measures. An alternative extreme approach aims at keeping the patient out of hospital as much as possible and away from the organisms that are particularly likely to colonize and cause serious infections in these patients. The most dangerous organisms in this respect are the hospital Gram-negative organisms, referred to above.

The value of oral non-absorbable antibiotics and protected environment in acute myeloblastic anaemia has been assessed in many studies [27]. In some [14, 28-30], but not all, the incidence of infection, days of infections, and incidence of fatal infections, at any neutrophil count have been reduced. Moreover, the remission in this disease has been improved, in some studies substantially [14, 27].

Granulocyte transfusions

It is now possible to treat patients with infection and neutropenia with granulocytes from a normal donor or from a patient with chronic granulocytic leukaemia. In general, granulocytes are only indicated for patients with neutrophil counts below $1.0 \times 10^9/1$ and fever over $38°C$ that has persisted for over 24 hours despite antibiotic therapy. Recent trials have unequivocally demonstrated the value of white cells prepared either by filtration-leucapheresis [31] or by continuous flow separation [32] in such patients. The therapy is most useful for patients with localized infection, if the transfusions contain more than 10^{10} leucocytes and if these can be repeated over several days [33-35]. Leucocytes from a patient with chronic granulocytic leukaemia, although not entirely normal functionally, are nevertheless of great value because of the large numbers that can be obtained. Occasionally, a chronic-granulocytic-leukaemia graft 'takes' in an immunosuppressed recipient but this is a temporary phenomenon lasting up to several weeks before the graft is rejected. A graft-versus-host reaction may also occur due to lymphocytes in the donated leucocytes and a fatal reaction, which must be extremely rare, has been reported [36]. This may be prevented by irradiation of the leucocytes with 1500 R which kills lymphocytes but leaves neutrophils functionally unimpaired. Granulocytes are collected by filtration leucapheresis or by a special continuous flow cell separator of the IMB or Aminco type or by discontinuous cell separation using the Haemonetic type of machine. Normal donors are given a single dose of steroid (e.g. dexamethasone) or aetiocholanione before donation to increase the number of circulating neutrophils, and hence the yield. In addition, with the use of cell separators, a sedimenting agent, e.g. hydroxyethyl starch, is given to the donor to improve separation of white cells from red cells. It is not usually possible to give HLA-matched granulocytes but, since granulocytes invariably contain a substantial number of red cells, it is preferable to give white cells from ABO-compatible donors. Although granulocytes collected by filtration leucapheresis show some impairment of function *in vitro* and are more prone to cause febrile reactions [37] they seem nearly as effective *in vivo* as those collected by a cell separator. Leucocytes in buffy coats obtained during preparation of platelet concentrates may also be useful (Figure 1). Although doubts have been cast on the functional

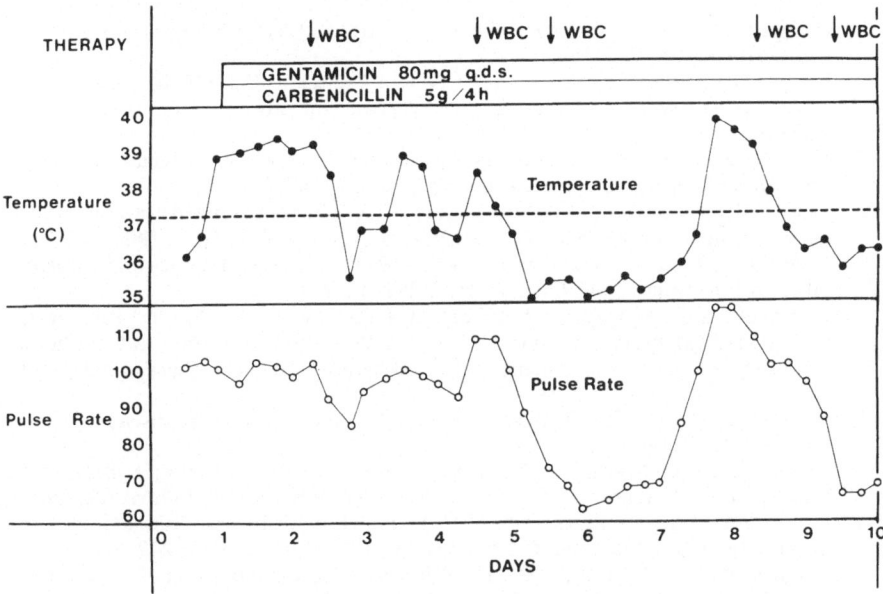

Figure 1. The response to buffy-coat white cells in a neutropenic patient (male aged 44) with acute myeloblastic leukaemia during remission induction. The patient had a neutrophil count less than $0.2 \times 10^9/l$ and developed fever which did not respond to antibiotics within 24 hours. No bacterial cause could be identified. A single infusion of leucocytes (2×10^{10}) produced a fall in temperature which was not sustained. Four further white-cell infusions, varying from 1×10^{10} to 5×10^{10}, produced further falls in temperature. After 10 days the patient's own neutrophil count rose to over $1.0 \times 10^9/l$ as the patient went into remission and the temperature remained normal.

efficiency of these concentrates, we have found them effective and use them regularly.

The most important aspect of whether or not granulocyte transfusion therapy is effective in infected neutropenic patients with acute leukaemia is recovery of bone-marrow function. It is quite remarkable how rapidly the most serious infection can subside once the bone-marrow recovers sufficiently to cause a rise in circulating granulocytes to over $1 \times 10^9/1$. On the other hand, in the absence of bone-marrow recovery, the outcome of severe infection in these patients despite antibiotics and granulocytes is often fatal.

References

1. Levine, A.S., Schimpff, S.C., Graw, R.G., and Young, R.C. (1974) Hematologic malignancies and other marrow failure states: progress in the management of complicating infections. *Sem. Hemat.*, **11**, 141–202
2. Gaya, H. (1975) The treatment of infection in acute leukaemia. *Br. J. Hosp. Med.* **13**, 124–129.
3. Bodey, G.P. (Ed) (1976) Infectious complications in haematological diseases. In *Clins. Haemat.* **5**, 227–469.
4. Bodey, G.P., Buckley, M., Sathe, Y.S. and Freireich, E.J. (1966) Quantitative relationships between circulating leucocytes and infection in patients with acute leukemia. *Ann. intern. Med.* **64**, 328–40.
5. Rodriguez, V. and Bodey, G.P. (1976) Antibacterial therapy—special considerations in neutropenic patients. *Clins. Haemat.*, **5**, 347–60.
6. Herzig, R.H., Poplack, D.G. and Yankee, R.A. (1974) Prolonged granulocytopenia from incompatible platelet transfusions. *New Engl. J. Med.* **290**, 1220–3.
7. Dale, D.C., Fauci, A.S. and Wolff, S.M. (1974) Leukocyte kinetics and susceptibility to infections. *New Engl. J. Med.* **291**, 1154–8.
8. Campbell, A.C., Hersey, P., MacLennan, I.C.M., Kay, H.E.M. and Pike, M.C. (1973) Medical Research Council Working Party on Leukaemia in Childhood. Immunosuppressive consequences of radiotherapy and chemotherapy in patients with ALL. *Br. med. J.* **2**, 385–8.
9. Valdivieso, M. (1976) Bacterial infection in haematological diseases. *Clins. Haemat.* **5**, 229–48.
10. Chang, H.Y., Rodriguez, V., Narboni, G., Bodey, G.P. and Freireich, E.J. (1975) Causes of death in adults with acute leukaemia. *Medicine Baltimore*, **55**, 256–8.
11. Krick, J.A. and Remington, J.S. (1976) Opportunistic invasive fungal infections in patients with leukaemia and lymphoma. *Clin. Haematol.* **5**, 249–310.
12. Hughes, W.T. and Smith, D.R. (1973) Infection during induction of remission in acute lymphocytic leukemia. *Cancer* **31**, 1008–14.
13. Rodriguez, V., Gutterman, J.U., McMullan, G.K. and Heckman, A.A. (1972) The spectrum of infections in patients with acute leukaemia and malignant lymphoma in a military hospital. *Military Med.* **137**, 199–202.
14. Levine, A.S., Siegel, S.E., Schreiber, A.D., Hauser, J., Preisler, H., Goldstein, F., Seidler, F., Simon, R., Perry, S., Bennett, J.E. and Henderson, E.J. (1973) Protected environments and prophylactic antibiotics. A prospective controlled study of their utility in the therapy of acute leukemia. *New Engl. J. Med.* **288**, 477–83.
15. Klastersky, J., Debusscher, L., Weerts, D. and Daneau, D. (1974) Use of oral antibiotics in protected environment units: clinical effectiveness and role in the emergence of antibiotic-resistant strains. *Path. Biol.* **22**, 5–12.
16. Feldman, S. and Cox, F, (1976) Viral infections and haematological malignancies. *Clins. Haematol.* **5**, 311–28.
17. Rodriguez, V., Burgess, M. and Bodey, G.P. (1973) Management of fever of unknown origin in patients with neoplasms and neutropenia. *Cancer* **32**, 1007–12.

18. Bodey, G.P., Middleman, E., Umsawasdi T., and Rodriguez, V. (1972) Infections in cancer patients: results with gentamicin sulfate therapy. *Cancer* **29**, 167–1701.
19. Smith, C.R., Baughman, K.L., Edwards, C.Q., Rogers, J.F., and Lietman, P.S. (1977) Controlled comparison of amikacin and gentamicin. *New Engl. J. Med.* **296**, 349–53.
20. Brown, C.H., Natelson, E.A., Bradshaw, M.W., Williams, T.W. Jr. and Alfrey, C.P. Jr. (1974) The hemostatic defect produced by carbenicillin. *New Engl. J. Med.* **291**, 265–70.
21. Kucers, A. and Bennett, N. McK. (1975) *The use of antibiotics. A comprehensive guide with clinical emphasis* 2nd edn, pp. 222. W. Heinemann Medical Books Ltd., London.
22. Gaya, H., Klastersky, J., Schimpff, S.C. and Tattersall, M.H.N. (1975) Protocol for an international prospective trial of initial therapy regimens in neutropenic patients with malignant disease. *Europ. J. Cancer* **1**. 1–4 (Suppl.).
23. Klastersky, J., Henri, A., Hensgens, C. and Daneau, D. (1974) Gram-negative infections in cancer. Study of empiric therapy comparing carbenicillin-cephalothin with and without gentamicin. *J. Am. Med. Ass.* **227**, 45–8.
24. Bodey, G.P., Chang, H.Y., Rodriguez, V. and Stewart, D. (1975) Feasibility of adminstering aminoglycoside antibiotics by continued intravenous infusion. *Antimicr. Ag. Chemother.* **8**, 328–33.
25. Bodey, G.P. and Rosenbaum, B. (1974) Effect of prophylactic measures on the microbial flora of patients in protected environment units. *Medicine Baltimore* **53**, 209–28.
26. Bodey, G.P. and Rodriguez, V. (1976) Protected environment—prophylactic antibiotic programmes; microbiological studies. *Clins. Haematol.* **5**, 395–408.
27. Levine, A.S. (1976) Protected environment—prophylactic antibiotic programmes; clinical studies. *Clins. Haematol.* **5**, 409–424.
28. Bodey, G.P. and Johnston (1971) Microbiological evaluation of protected environments during patient occupancy. *Appl. Microbiol.* **22**, 828–36.
29. Yates, J.W. and Holland, J.F. (1973) A controlled study of isolation and endogenous microbial suppression in acute myelocytic leukemia patients. *Cancer* **32**, 1490–8.
30. Schimpff, S.C., Greene, W.H., Young, V.M., Fortner, C.L., Jepsen, L., Cusak, N., Block, J.B. and Wiernik, P.H. (1975) Infection prevention in acute non-lymphocytic leukemia: laminar air-flow room reverse isolation with oral, non-absorbable antibiotic prophylaxis. *Ann. int. Med.* **82**, 351–8.
31. Higby, D.J., Yates, J.W., Henderson, E.S. and Holland, J.F. (1975) Filtration leukapheresis for granulocyte transfusion therapy. *New Engl. J. Med.* **292**, 761–6.
32. Herzig, R.H., Herzig, G.P., Graw, R.G., Bull, M.I. and Ray, K.K. (1977) Granulocyte transfusion therapy for Gram-negative septicemia. *New Engl. J. Med.* **296**, 701–5.
33. Graw, R.G. Jr., Herzig, G., Perry, S. and Henderson, E.S. (1972) Normal granulocyte transfusion therapy. Treatment of septicemia due to gram-negative bacteria. *New Engl. J. Med.* **287**, 367–71.
34. Lowenthal, R.M., Grossman, L., Goldman, J.M., Storring, R.A., Buskard, N.A., Park, D.S., Murphy, B.C., Spiers, A.S.D. and Galton, D.A.G. (1975) Granulocyte transfusions in treatment of infections in patients with acute leukaemia and aplastic anaemia. *Lancet* i, 353–61.
35. Alavi, J.B., Root, R.K., Djerassi, I., Evans, A.E., Gluckman, S.J., MacGregor, R.R., Guerry, D., Schreiber, A.D., Shaw, J.M., Koch, P. and Cooper, R.A. (1977) Clinical trial of granulocyte transfusions for infection in acute leukemia. *New Engl. J. Med.* **296**, 706–11.
36. Ford, J.M., Cullen, M.H., Lucey, J.J., Tobias, J.S. and Lister, T.A. (1976) Fatal graft-versus-host disease following transfusion of granulocytes from normal donors. *Lancet* ii, 1167–9.

37. Herzig, G.P., Root, R.K. and Graw, R.G. (1972) Granulocyte collection by continuous flow filtration leukapheresis. *Blood,* **39**, 554–67.

Discussion

Dr. Wallace: I am not sure of the value of monitoring once a week. Can you explain its purpose and tell me what do you do when you find organisms that may be pathogenic?

Prof. Hoffbrand: If we find staphylococci or a Gram-negative organism on the skin surfaces or in noses we tend to treat with local antiseptics in an attempt to eliminate them. In general, the patients' infections come from themselves or from people in contact with them.

Dr. Noone: We look particularly for *Pseudomonas aeruginosa*, yeasts and other multi-resistant organisms in these patients. There is good evidence from the Hammersmith that if you find patients with psuedomonads on their person or in their bowel, you really must do something about it. If you leave it this will almost certainly progress to a systemic infection.

Dr. Wallace: What about the lungs? One so often finds coliforms in sputum.

Dr. Noone: First of all one has to decide whether it is coming from the lung or just from the patient's pharynx. If it is in the pharynx, this can be quite useful information as it can progress from there to become a serious infection.

Dr. Wallace: How would you treat a coliform in the pharynx?

Dr. Noone: A pseudomonad will often be removed by oral colistin. It is also worthwhile checking on the flora of the nursing staff and others in contact with the patients. If patients are found to be contaminated with hospital organisms, this suggests that there has been a breakdown in the reverse isolation procedures.

Dr. Lal: When you take action, you are going to take an important step in the management of the patient. Do you act when there is either leucopenia or fever, and would you take action on the strength of a single positive blood culture?

Prof. Hoffbrand: The criterion should be neutropenia and fever, or, a local lesion and neutropenia. Clearly fever by itself is a worrying symptom but the usual problem is a combination of neutropenia and fever. The threshold for severe danger of neutropenia is now regarded as less than 100 per cubic millimetre. Patients with 500 neutrophils per cubic millimetre are now considered to be well off, despite the lower limit for normals of 1500. However, many of the patients that we see have virtually no neutrophils, and any of them developing a fever (a temperature of 100° F or greater) will be treated. The trouble with blood cultures is that results do not come for several days, by which time we have had to start treatment. If the organism isolated is one which we are not covering, we change treatment.

Dr. Hobson: I was interested in the difference you found between leukaemics and patients with Hodgkin's disease in susceptibility to infection. Are there differences in white cell function? Is this due to the different cytotoxic regime given, or could it perhaps be correlated with differences in the antibody response or in cell-mediated immunity?

Prof. Hoffbrand: Patients with leukaemia are deficient in both phago-cytes and monocytes. In skin-window experiments, patients with Hodgkin's disease are better able to mobilize neutrophils to the skin windows than are leukaemics. There may be low neutrophil counts due to other conditions such as hypersplenism, but there is bone-marrow reserve in Hodgkin's, which there is not in acute leukaemia. In addition, I think you are quite right in suggesting that there is a functional deficiency in neutrophils in leukaemics. For instance, their myeloperoxidase is often decreased.

Prof. Asscher: I would like to ask Prof. Hoffbrand about fever being used as his sole criterion. In Cardiff, a sudden drop of blood pressure is regarded as an important indication of a serious infection. What do you think the pathogenesis of fever is in patients with low white-cell counts?

Prof. Hoffbrand: Pyrogens must be coming from sources other than white cells. By and large fever is a pretty good indication and most leukaemic patients who become infected develop fever. However, you are right that it is not 100%. We could not withhold treatment with antibiotics merely because the patient was afebrile but for practical purposes fever must be taken as the main indication.

Prof. Asscher: In renal units Gram-negative septicaemia may occur with no fever at all, just hypotension. I was very interested to hear that this was not so in leukaemics.

Prof. Brumfitt: I would like to raise two matters. First, the fact that gentamicin by itself does not work in leukaemics. At a recent interna-tional meeting on aminoglycosides, Dr. Noone mentioned that results were less satisfactory in respiratory infections and in this connection we have found (*The Lancet*, 1976) that the aminoglycosides work less well under a reduced oxygen tension. Do you think that one of the reasons why gentamicin does not work is that due to accompanying anaemia oxygen tension in the tissues is reduced? Secondly, the question of progressive colonization. When we first started doing kidney transplantation at St. Mary's, we were plagued by pseudomo-nas infection. It was very characteristic to observe patients getting positive throat swabs and rectal swabs on routine swabbing, followed by urinary tract infection spreading to the kidney, resulting in death. This was greatly reduced not by reverse isolation, but simply by decreasing the amount of immunosuppressive agent. It was titrated so as to increase the patient's resistance to what is, after all, a rather weak pathogen.

Prof. Hoffbrand: The activity of gentamicin in neutropenic patients seems to depend upon the neutrophil count, irrespective of other aspects such as anaemia and severity of underlying disease. Gentamicin is bactericidal in patients with very few neutrophils, and there are obviously several possible explanations for this. The difficulty with acute myeloid leukaemia is that the drugs used for treating it are toxic to the bone marrow (as they do not differentiate between normal and diseased cells). The newer antileukaemic regimes tend to be more toxic and aggressive and they cause more profound neutropenia and immunosuppression. The aim of treatment in many series is to cause bone-marrow aplasia, to support the patient, and hope that they will grow normal cells. So I am afraid that there seems to be very little hope of leukaemic experts producing less immunosuppression. In patients over 50 with acute leukaemia—who tend to do extremely badly—there may be a tendency not to use such aggressive therapy, however.

Dr. Tones: Do you have a problem with anaerobes?

Prof. Hoffbrand: I am not aware that, over the past two years, many of our patients have had septicaemias or local lesions diagnosed as being due to anaerobic bacteria.

Dr. Noone: Some leukaemic patients have had problems with anaerobes. I can remember at least two patients extremely ill with anaerobic infection who had fistula-in-ano. They responded to metronidazole.

Prof. Hoffbrand: There is a difference between local lesions and patients dying of anaerobic septicaemias. Obviously some are going to be colonizing their local lesion from the gut.

Dr. Willis: I was a bit surprised that anaerobes other than clostridia did not figure at all. Is this because they were not looked for or they did not cause death in terms of septicaemia? Gram-negative anaerobes are the commonest organisms in the body and in compromised patients they are a common cause of septicaemia. Carbenicillin covers most of these anaerobes and I wonder if the greatly improved effect of carbenicillin and gentamicin may be attributable to inhibition of anaerobes?

Prof. Hoffbrand: I suppose it depends on the ability of the laboratory to grow anaerobes. Some of the infections we see are multiple: in some series as many as a fifth of all the septicaemias are due to more than one organism. We have had remarkably few septicaemias in which anaerobes have been grown from blood cultures.

Dr. Selwyn: I just wondered if we could look briefly at the question of isolation and decontamination. We are lucky to have a couple of Trexler isolators, in which patients feel very happy. They are not cut off. Children can be cuddled by their mother and the nurses do not have to wear special clothing. That's one thing we like and we want to get more of these. The other thing, on decontamination, I think it is very wrong to use nystatin to try to get rid of yeasts. We failed miserably, and we are now using amphotericin B because we and Dutch workers have shown a prolonged effect with this compound. In the mouth there are considerable problems of decontamination. We are now using Obrabase which is a material in which any antibiotic can be incorporated. This gives a prolonged release of the antibiotic, and now we are able to approach the problem of oral decontamination with much greater confidence.

Index